PRESENCE, PROFICIENT, PROFESSIONAL

An Executive Guide to Exude
Confidence and Distinction

Agnes Koh

Founder of Etiquette & Image International
President of The Etiquette Alliance International

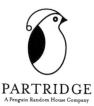

PARTRIDGE
A Penguin Random House Company

To order additional copies of this book, contact
Toll Free 800 101 2657 (Singapore)
Toll Free 1 800 81 7340 (Malaysia)
orders.singapore@partridgepublishing.com

www.partridgepublishing.com/singapore

Table of Contents

Introduction

Presence | Proficient | Professional

A little child loves your presence and not your presents. Everyone has a degree of childlike needs inside us. When you are with somebody, you crave his attention. It is an invisible warmth that can be felt immediately. It is a close communication of earthiness and comfort he provides.

According to Albert Mebrabian, Professor Emeritus of Psychology, UCLA, widely known for his findings on the messages of feelings, attitudes and human communication, presence consists of the 7%-38%-55% rule:

7%—Verbal Communication
38%—Vocal Communication
55%—Visual Communication

In today's practical world, you are being judged on presence. This includes non-verbal communication of your looks, dress, hairstyle, as well as verbal communication of your voice, words and behaviour. Quite simply, perception is not real, but it does impact how you affect the subconscious of others.

A pleasant image contributes your growth and progress. Your first impression determines your business advantage. It is an influential edge to attract the right people, ace your interviews or run a leadership role. Like it or not, if you carry a poised image, confident and well mannered, you instantly win people with your ideas because you are worthy of trust, approachable and respectable; that is proficient.

Your image is priceless. It is strongly affected by your self-assurance, how you portray your personal credentials and your social approach to network building as a basis for achieving business success in Asia.

Lastly, adhering to ethical and moral values is an honourable course of deserving esteem and respect in the business arena. Be professional and do not ruin it.

The Importance of Good Etiquette

How others perceive you is an often overlooked thing. The "I don't care" attitude will only take you so far, but it will not move you up the likeability chart.

Etiquette is like a mirror. It reflects on your civility, upbringing and wisdom. Etiquette has become a way of life and a ticket to bridge a harmonious relationship and prevent offences.

We have all heard of that one person who did something in front of the right people that led to a deal being cancelled and ultimately ruined his chances in the company. This could happen to almost anyone.

At your workplace, just because you have worked for years in a company does not mean that you are top dog and are the closest to a promotion. When moving up the corporate ladder, your skills are not the only skills that are considered. Alvin Toffler, an American writer and futurist, once stated, 'The illiterate of the 21st century will not be those who cannot read and write, but those who cannot learn, unlearn, and relearn." Toffler is also frequently cited as stating, "Tomorrow's illiterate will not be the man who can't read; he will be the man who has not learned how to learn."

You can't buy a genuine social or business relationship, though you may have a high-flying paper qualification. It is important to sustain decent, socially accepted behaviour and keep the bridge. Some of your behaviours are a reflection of your family upbringing and along the way, you may wish to unlearn your attitude and relearn a new way to improve a relationship.

How to Acquire Good Business Etiquette

A quick way to learn good business etiquette is from a person directly. This would, however, require that you to gain the trust of the person first. The best way to approach the situation is with an honest and sincere attitude and when the time is right, request some help. Observe and take note of your company's CEO or a department manager. There is no safer way to learn good business etiquette than to observe it firsthand and learn from them.

One final way is to pick up various books like this one and learn in a simple, concise and less time consuming way on how to attain good business etiquette.

The Asian Culture

The Asian culture is more sensitive to business etiquette than any other market. This is not because of weird and obscure reasons as many people tend to think, but it is very closely tied to Asian's socio-economic cultural diversity.

Many western representatives from various companies who visit Asian countries to sell their product, close a deal or personally deal with a business issue have gone back empty-handed because they were impatient, direct and outspoken, and this developed into an impolite gesture or comment in their business meeting.

Agnes Koh

The Aim of This Book

This book provides an accelerated return on your investment. My most effective techniques from a diverse experience of Etiquette, Image, Fitness, Health and Wellness disciplines. My aim is to allow you to apply immediately, gain merit for yourself and support your proficiency and knowledge. So explore and extract those skills, suggestions and techniques you can easily put into practice.

Not only is this book detailed, it is very simple to understand, using informative text combined with pictures.

Regardless of whether you are a fresh graduate looking for an edge, or if you are a long-term employee who has not earned your rightful due, this book will help you attain heights that you may never have thought could be reached.

Lastly, do put it into practice to yield its full benefits. Your patience and resilience to apply what you read and see it through is your pinnacle.

Chapter One

Appearances, Grooming, Health, Well-being and Proper Business Attire

Appearances Are Everything

Presentable

The Merriam-Webster dictionary defined "presentable" as being in good condition (not messy, dirty, unclean) before others, especially by the critical. Outward appearances mean a lot in the business world. In less than 10 seconds, we subconsciously form a perception about others based on visual "evidence".

My Personal Testimonial

I entered the hospitality industry at a tender age of 19. It was every young girl's dream to be in a glamorous job. At 5 feet, 1 inch tall, I was unable to pursue being a flight stewardess with Singapore Airlines. I decided to explore hospitality on the "ground". In the early 90s, the choices were Manufacturing or Service Industry in Singapore's developing business climate. I had the proudest moment among my classmates when I joined The Westin Stamford & Westin Plaza Singapore.

Coming from a big family, we had to make our own survival bowl upon finishing school. I only had one basic need in mind at that time—FREE FOOD in order to save some expenses for night classes.

Agnes Koh

The Blue Suit

Reminiscing over my job interview, I had my brand-new navy blue suit, 2 and a half inch heels with nude hosiery and light makeup comprised of foundation powder and a sweet rosy lipstick.

I went through the typing proficiency test and two interviews with the HR Manager and Director, respectively. The final interview was with the Food & Beverage Director and hearing his name made me nervous. At 6 feet tall, this humongous German was famous for his strict discipline on staff grooming. He took a quick glance at me when I stood up after the interview. I still felt small as he walked me out of the door, shook my hand, introduced me to his secretary I would be working with and said, "Welcome aboard."

Real Live Experience

The management and staff offered their finest service to make sure guests had their best memory during their stay. Hence, the practice of good etiquette, emotional quotient, relationship, rapport and mingling skills came 'live' as a package.

The exciting and glamorous experience afforded me opportunities to embark on more than a decade of career advancements. Each day was different from the previous. New challenges increased as I moved up the ladder from F&B Catering to Sales in many deluxe chain hotels. Naturally, I focused on creating the best first impression for every guest's stay with us.

The Poise Industry

The cruel fact in the front line was they would hesitate to hire an overweight employee because the perception of that person was more often "plump", "slow" and "fat." Employees who were slender were perceived as presentable, educated, sociable and friendly.

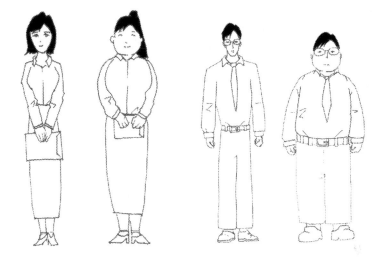

Which lady would you choose?   Which man would you choose?

A poll conducted randomly on 50 women by *Women's Weekly* in November 2011, 96% of respondents said women who are slender are perceived as presentable, presence, proficient and friendly.

In no way are we telling you to work towards six-pack abs, but at least have a sleek, healthy and slim body.

Healthy Body, Healthy Mind

The ironic part of being a hotelier was you enjoyed great food, wine and dine at posh outlets. I noticed my waist had gone horizontal. I realized that my increased stress level, long hours and great demand for physical presence at the hotel kept me away from exercise.

I had no time for hobbies, interests or activities outside my work until I landed a regional job as Sales & Marketing Manager for an overseas hotel. Life became normal, from 9-6 pm, and I started working out in the gym. I joined group exercise classes and developed an interest in teaching aerobics. I signed up for a 3-month intensive training to certify myself as a trainer, started teaching regularly and found a new passion.

When you look pleasant on the outside, you will automatically feel rewarded on the inside. They say a sound body goes hand in hand with a healthy mind, and millions of wellness experts obviously cannot be wrong.

Good physical health will not only help you feel and perform better at work, it will also help improve your personal and work life.

When I joined Planet Hollywood in 2000 as Sales & Marketing Manager, the all-star theme café chain had me exuberant. It was a dining experience inspired by the glamour and excitement of the big screen and featuring an extensive Hollywood memorabilia collection, including props from blockbuster movies and classic TV shows. At that time, I was teaching fitness classes three times a week. I was so liberated and enjoyed going back to office after an hour of teaching and had never felt any drag at all. My life revolved around committing to the love-of-my life, and I had never felt so happy.

Regular exercise combats persistent fatigue, stress, depression, and mood swings. Exercise releases endorphins, energy cells and neurotransmitters to the brain. This principle is perhaps the reason I stay energized.

A healthy mind helps to keep your body moving in an optimum condition. The confidence helps you improve the quality of your work and allows you to work better and faster.

If you are wondering how good physical health improves your work life, I am the living proof. When you are physically fit, you feel proficient and that reflects in your inter-office relations and the quality of your work.

Today, working out at the local gym is convenient. Going for a daily jog in the park is a very easy way to attain a healthy body and better well-being. Joining your workplace exercise programs or a quick half-hour treadmill are also great ways to get a work-life balance.

You may have a pet that you rarely take out for walks and usually get someone else to do. Take yourself and your dog out for a walk. Not only is it good for him/her, it is also very therapeutic for you.

Every human being requires adequate rest and nutrition. Develop good eating habits of three meals a day. The ancient Chinese Proverb says, "A good breakfast cannot be replaced by the evening meal." It is important to eat a balanced diet of 4-5 small meals a day to avoid unhealthy cravings. In addition, multiple small meals will help to keep you full all day. However, food should consist of lots of vegetables, fruits, white meat and the occasional slab of red meat.

The KCB Diet

Another ancient Chinese quote states, "Eat good breakfast like a King, moderate lunch like a Civilian and very light dinner like a Beggar." The KCB diet is one in which food intake reduces gradually from day to night. A detailed explanation is given below.

Eat Breakfast like a King

The most important meal of the day is breakfast. Many working executives skip breakfast in the attempt to lose weight or sleep in for few more minutes or to avoid the morning rush to work, etc.

With a low blood-sugar level, the brain does not work optimally. Research at the UT Southern Medical Centre by Dr Jeffrey

Zigman, assistant professor of internal medicine and psychiatry, found that hunger hormones called ghrelin are obstructed.

Ghrelin affects many behavioural responses that correspond to appetite, hunger pangs, mood, stress and energy levels. Some ideal choices of food group, according to "The Food Doctor", include whole-meal pasta, oatmeal, toasted muesli, wheat, sourdough rye, multigrain porridge, wholegrain bread.

Lunch like a Civilian

Eat a moderate lunch that contains soupy meals. However, avoid fried food at all costs. People who skip breakfast usually eat more at lunch and snack throughout the day.

The release of ghrelin is transmitted repeatedly to the brain, requesting it to cover the loss of breakfast, making you feel hungrier for longer, despite the recent meal.

Making the wrong food choices will lead to weight gain, especially when you take into account the almost stationery nature of most office work. You will feel very lethargic after lunch, and this will negatively affect your concentration during office hours.

Eat Dinner like a Beggar

Most people eat dinner and then go to sleep. This immobility after eating unfortunately leads to the build-up of body fat while you sleep. This is why it is best to keep dinner light. A light dinner results in less fat accumulation during sleep.

Even sitting in front of the television or computer will increase body fat, as you are immobile. For dinner, try sandwiches, salad or fruits to prevent the craving for food and disturbing your sleep.

If you are paying attention to the process of eating, the most effective way to maintain a healthy weight is to consume fewer calories as the day ends. If you embark on a weight loss regime, the effective way is to have your dinner before 5pm and acquire a habit of not eating before bedtime.

Exercise—Use it or Lose it

Have you heard the expression "use it or lose it?" The enormous benefits of exercise can only be reaped when you move your body. When you exercise, you improve your stamina, strengthen your heart and tone your muscles. It prevents diseases and controls your weight. It improves your flexibility and endurance level. On the contrary, if you do not use your body, you will lose those abilities cited above, and your joints and muscles will suffer deleterious effects. You lose your lean tissue, and your limited energy will drain off eventually.

Fitness for Life

Do you "exercise to get fit or get fit to exercise?" The former refers to a state of well-being and sustaining a healthy lifestyle, whereas the latter refers to a specific goal to achieve and maintain. Many people tend to compromise or stop completely after they have achieved a fitness goal. Maintenance of your lifestyle does not mean you have to religiously follow through a 100% schedule. Do not slide into the old habits or relapse. It is lifestyle maintenance.

Always build your exercise regime with the following 5 components:

1. **Cardiovascular Fitness**—Jogging, swimming, cycling, dancing or aerobic exercise to deliver oxygen to your muscles and improve your heart and lung function.

2. **Muscular Strength**—Light weightlifting to condition and define the muscle groups and eliminate fat.

3. **Muscular Endurance**—Pilates, Yoga and other conditioning exercises work on muscular endurance. It is the ability to repeat a movement or isolate a particular pose for an extended period.

4. **Flexibility**—Pilates & Yoga help to lengthen and relax the muscles.

5. **Body Composition**—Always check your body fat compared to the amount of lean mass (muscle, bones, etc.).

Exercise at least three times a week for optimal health. Make a list of how important a fitness routine is to you when you fall into comfort food rituals. Watch what you eat when you have an event or celebration, we do not condone over-emphasising your restriction in the presence of your friends, where bonding takes priority at times.

Adequate Rest and Nutrition

Adequate rest helps nourish your body and renew your glandular cells. The benefits of sleep affect every area of our life.

The Benefits of Good Sleep

Our immune system (lymphatic system) retreats into an auto-detoxification and cells are renewed between 9pm and 11pm. You should be relaxing both your brain and body. You may practice deep breathing to calm your autonomous nerves and emotions. Listening to some soothing music will ease away the tension and prepare you for a calming state.

Your liver starts to auto-cleanse when you go into deep sleep between 11pm and 3pm. We all know the liver is the most important organ, as its function is to eliminate wastes and toxins from the body. Hence, it is not advisable to consume any alcoholic drinks before bed time.

Your gallbladder, lungs and large intestines will purge out impurities between 3am and 7am. If you cough or have a bowel movement, the organs evacuate poisonous microorganisms.

Lastly, the small intestines absorb the maximum nutrients between 7am and 9am, so you should not skip breakfast. The KCB Diet works very well.

> *Tips to promote good sleep*
>
> *Fight against late nights, chronic fatigue and insomnia with doses of minerals such as magnesium, Vitamin D, B, A, Beta-carotene, C, Zinc and Coenzyme Q10. These minerals can be found in vegetables such as celery, cauliflower, spinach, garlic, romaine lettuce, carrots, cabbage, broccoli and soybeans.*

Personal Grooming

Hygiene

Hygiene is of the utmost importance when it comes to keeping up appearances. Take a few factors into consideration and be honest with yourself.

- Would you talk to someone with bad breath?

- Would you shake hands with a colleague who forgot to wash his hands after using the bathroom or eating a meal?

- Would you come near a colleague who forgot to shower (evident by bad body odour)

The answer to all those questions is a definite no. It does not matter whether you are with or without someone, it is crucial to maintain good hygiene.

As an example, brushing your teeth in the morning will not only give you fresh breath but a confident smile. Bad breath turns away people and gives displeasure to your prospects if you are working in customer service.

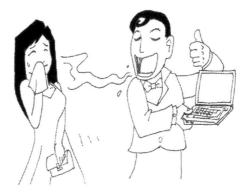

Clean hands and even good body odour go a long way and also instil self-confidence. Good hygiene will give you an inviting aura in the work place and will definitely give you a huge confidence boost. People will enjoy being with you and working with you closely.

When it comes to hygiene, it is always good to have more information. Personal hygiene is the maintenance of personal cleanliness and sanitation of the body. Some extra points include:

- Bathe daily, as this will eliminate body odour. Apply anti-perspirant or deodorant.

- If you smoke, polish your teeth regularly. Invest in a home bleaching tool kit. In addition, always keep some breath mints with you.

- Carry a tube of toothpaste and a toothbrush with you and make it a habit to brush your teeth after each meal.

- Dry eyes can produce a crusty spot around the corner of the eyes. To avoid this problem, clean your eyes regularly. If you have a problem with dry eyes, visit an ophthalmologist who may prescribe eye drops.

- Never dig in your nose or ear in public. This is a very unsightly gesture. Most people grow their last fingernail for this purpose, and it should never be done.

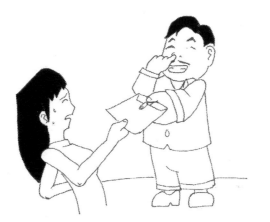

- Do not pick your pimples, scabs or dry warts.

- Trim your extra or unwanted facial hair and make it a weekly habit. Be sure to keep your beard and/or goatee neat and trimmed and keep your 5 o'clock shadow constantly checked.

- Exfoliate your skin and feet weekly or at least once a month. The frequency varies from your exposure in the environment, your lifestyle and work nature.

- It is essential to trim your finger and toe nails.

- Never break wind in public and think you can get away un-noticed. If you do not wish to be labelled as the "toxic colon person", do not do it in public.

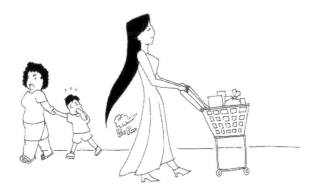

- Do not expect others to maintain eye contact when you lift up your arms to scratch your armpit or even aerate your underarms. If you ever need to do any of these things, do it in a bathroom and thoroughly wash your hands afterwards.

- Avoid bra straps that slip from your shoulders. Most women spend time fixing the straps throughout the day and it can make the person talking to you feel uncomfortable. Try wearing a strapless bra and combining it with a spaghetti top.

- Being bald may look good on many people but the extra fertilized patch that can grow needs to be trimmed to finish and maintain the look.

- Always press all your clothes and never go to work with an article of clothing that has not been pressed.

- Polish your shoes before you step out of the house.

- For those wearing glasses, always keep them clean. Smudge marks and scratches not only look awkward, they also hinder your view.

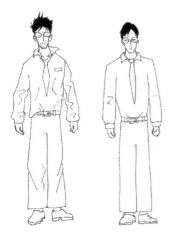

Difference between kempt and unkempt

Posture

Having good posture plays a vital part in your deportment. Slouching makes you look shorter and bone idle.

Acquire a habit of always standing in an upright position. If you do not know what this means, imagine a pen is inserted vertically between your naval and your heart.

Erect your spinal cord and keep both sides of your torso straight rather than bent on one side. Broaden your collar bones and engage the "wings" of your upper back to open up your chest. Keep your arms relaxed along your sides.

A slouched posture sends out a visual cue of being unproductive, moody, emotional and restless. Your poor posture will have a negative impact on your leadership. Good posture will always instil more confidence in your steps.

Shoddy Postures Kill Your Image

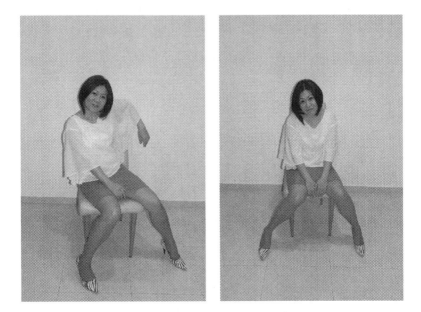

Dispositional attributes of Confident and Poised Postures

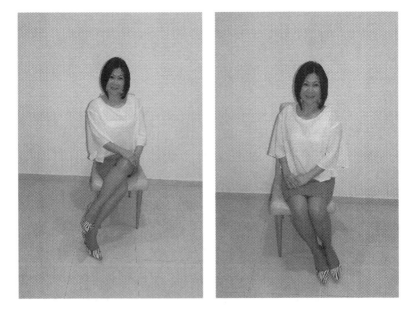

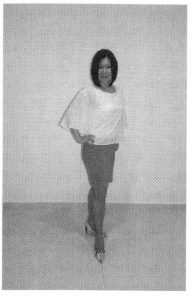

A tall standing posture—good
for taking portrait

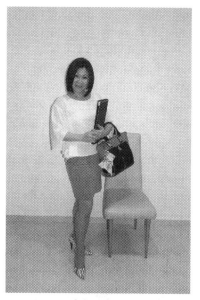

A graceful posture when
you have belongings

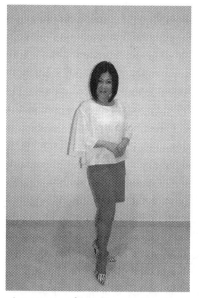

A posture of readiness when you
are speaking with someone

Walk Confidently

When wearing heels, you should walk by pointing your toes straight ahead instead of turning them out. Do not drag your feet but rather set your heel first, before the ball. Keep your legs parallel and swing your right arm as you step with your left foot and left arm as you step with your right foot to maintain balanced weight distribution on both sides. Always walk with your head erect without protruding the neck forward and never bend your body. As has been previously stated, confidence is a key factor, and keep the energy level up at all times.

Skin

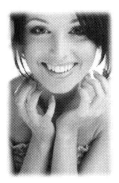

One often overlooked aspect of a person's physical appearance is the skin. Maintenance has often been perceived as a feminine area and men usually kept their distance. It was mainly due to the reduced macho nature that kept men at bay.

However, times have changed concerning beauty regimes for both men and women. Although skin maintenance is more important for women, men are also required to make a few changes to their skin. This is extremely crucial with a humid climate in Asia.

Some skin care tips include:

- Have sufficient sleep of at least 8 hours. Cells renewal starts from 11pm and continues till 2am.

- After your shower, apply toner to your face and the excess on your arms and legs to smoothen out the appearance of dull skin.

- Do not smoke, as the harmful tobacco not only affects the lungs; the nicotine wrinkles your eyes and mouth and makes your skin drier and sallow.

- If you have oily skin, use an astringent to restrict the overproduction of oil by the sebaceous oil glands. This will help keep your pores clean. Always use products with PH balanced formulae to control your T-zone and keep other parts of your face moisturized.

- Seek a dermatologist if you have signs of regular Papules (small solid rounded bumps, often pink in colour), as they can eventually develop into medium or large pustules.

- Keep the pores free from blockages by having a facial done at least once a month. Unclogging is usually done using a manual extraction method. Use high-frequency impulse light to reduce the appearance of wrinkles, uneven pigmentation and acne.

- Rejuvenate your skin with six professional steps in a salon: cleansing, exfoliation, massage, masking and moisturizing. These six actions will help keep your skin youthful, healthy and clear.

- Avoid fat-rich fried foods and food with high sugar content, such as chocolates and sweets.

- Have lots of greens, fruits, vitamin C and E, minerals selenium, copper and iron and drink at least two litres of water daily. Alternatively, drink 2 glasses of water in the morning to activate internal organs, 1 glass of water before showering to lower blood pressure and 1 glass of water at least two hours before bedtime to calm the heart and nerves.

4 such bottle sizes are equivalent to 2 litres.

- Dehydration leads to poor blood circulation, causing the blood vessels in the eyes, face and neck to dry, and lines look much more noticeable. When you are hydrated, you are less likely to develop dark circles underneath the eyes and uneven skin tone.

- Avoid going in the sun a lot and if you need to, use sun screen marked with at least a broad spectrum SPF30 / PA+++ (UVA, UVB).

- Ultraviolet radiation dramatically dries your skin, causing free radicals and freckles to develop. Hence, always avoid any UV radiation.

- If skin is not kept fresh, it loses its glow and shows its age. Moisturize your skin within 3 minutes after a bath. This helps to seal the richness of the moisturizer and achieve maximum results.

- Get some activity. Do not sit at your desk for hours. Immobility affects your blood circulation. The long hours at your desktop are detrimental to your eyes and facial skin.

- Enjoy and do little things in life for one day, you will look back and realize they were the big things—Robert Bravlt.

Tips to promote skin cell growth and reproduction

A simple recipe that you can prepare at home: 1 sliced of pineapple (cut into chunks), 1 mango (pitted), 1 peeled cucumber. Blend the pineapple,

followed by mango and cucumber. Squeeze the lemon and stir before serving. The cucumber has a trace mineral called silica to strengthen connective tissues. It reduces water retention and is high in Vitamins A, B, C and folic acid.

Anti-aging tips—Dermatologists' Recommendation

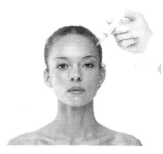

What were once considered to be stigmas are now as normal as getting your hair trimmed. These normal procedures help to keep the skin glowing and youthful. Most people, however, cannot find the right dermatologist, and the fact is they should not have to.

Ask a friend who has had the below recommendations done. Word of mouth is usually better than casual Internet research. In addition, you should always ask your dermatologist details about the procedure and its accompanying side effects and possible complications.

A few of the most common recommendations include:

Intense Pulse Light (IPL)—a photo-rejuvenation treatment that lightens age spots, freckles, broken capillaries, birthmarks and reduces pore size for a flawless complexion.

Chemical Peels—A treatment where chemical solution is applied to exfoliate dead cells and eliminate black/white heads, blemishes, acne scars, and pigmentation for a smoother and clearer complexion.

Laser Procedures—remove birthmarks, moles, spider veins, broken capillaries, warts, and other blemishes.

Botox—micro injections of purified protein relax and paralyze the facial muscles to correct and prevent wrinkles. In today's beauty world, Botox injection does not carry the mortification behind the scene anymore. Women are using it casually as part of their overall maintenance and grooming routine, much like a visit to the nail or hair salon.

Fillers—collagen or Hyaluronic Acid dermal fillers are injected to fill up deep wrinkles, furrows, hollow cheeks and to reshape the chin, jaw and nose bridge for a youthful look.

Crowning Glory

In the image perception chart, your looks account for 55% of who you are (apart from face). Next is your hair, hairstyle and finally nails. There are differences in male and female grooming but its necessity is the same for both sexes.

Fashionable yet Professional Office Hairstyles for Females

When you start talking to a colleague, boss or friend, 90% of a person's focus is redirected from the chest to the head. Taking this fact into consideration, you need to keep your facial appearance professional.

Your hairstyle should be appropriate and harmonize with your work attire and your corporate environment. It is understandable that a ponytail is quite boring but that does not mean you come to work every day with a fun hairstyle. Your image has to be both understated and elegant.

The following hairstyles are perfect for work. They are simple, require minimal effort to style and look smart and competent at the same time.

The Business Bun

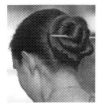

A business bun is chic yet sophisticated hairstyle and best of all, requires less than five minutes of your precious morning time to create. Simply part your hair on one side and gather your hair into a low ponytail. Twist the ponytail around the base and secure the bun with bobby pins.

The hair bun maker is a handy accessory to have. It is a round dough sponge that is used as an anti-slip tool for creating neat buns. It is a worthy investment for any woman. Follow these steps:

1. Secure your hair on the top or back of your head by using a ponytail band or hand grip

2. Swiftly pull your hair through the bun

3. Grip a small portion of your hair and arrange it around the bun until it is completely covered and secure with bobby pins

4. You can also use some light hair spray to secure the bun. This will help prevent unwanted loose strands for many hours. This step is optional yet highly recommended

Pixie hairstyles

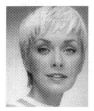

A short stylish haircut shows confidence and attitude. Short haircuts portray a strong personality and an assertive character. In fact, short hair gives people the impression that you are a hardworking, energetic and sharp person.

Short hairstyles such as the pixie style, however, demand regular maintenance. Although a little time consuming, they exude a personality unlike any other and will truly set you apart from other colleagues. The best part is that pixie styles are exceptionally versatile. As an example, you could spike the style up with some gel or mousse and go from corporate elite to "party animal" look in seconds.

Bob Hairstyles

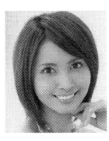

Bob hairstyles are classic and fashion forward. In fact, bobs can be of different variations, styles and cuts that help them suit any face shape. The varieties include short, mid-length and less puffy bobs. Believe it or not, when you cut a bob style in a salon, do not cross your legs and throw off your alignment the next time you wish for even results.

Many celebrities wear beautiful and trendy bobs. Victoria Beckham got the crowd moving by adopting a bob as her signature hairstyle.

Bob hairstyles are easy to maintain, work well with many hair textures and also enhance various facial features. Of all the other hairstyles mentioned, it is the easiest to maintain and does not necessitate any accessory or any extra styling—it is appropriate for any occasion.

If you have fine and thin hair, you might be unable to achieve a concave effect of the bob. Get a volumnizing shampoo. It is known for creating glamorous and fuller texture. Alternatively, dry shampoo is a great way to make the fine hair look fuller. Avoid shampoo that comes with conditioners, they have little moisturizing effect and weigh your hair down.

The Ideal Haircut for Men

Most mid-twenties individuals should know by now that their haircut is a reflection of their lifestyle. It would look weird if your boss came to work on Monday morning with a quirky and wild haircut. This is because every type of hairstyle has its age limits and creates varied impressions. The same applies to senior members.

Likewise, a young, fresh and Mohawk-style haircut may look good to many, but he will never look professional. Again, nobody will take you seriously if you come to work with such a haircut. The problem is that the current highly individual generation loves to keep up with the latest trends. When they enter the workplace, they have trendy hairstyles, which may appease similar colleagues, but they will never be taken seriously by senior workers.

Men with long hair come off as free-spirited and adventurous which, although it may seem acceptable in a creative industry, does not seem so in a corporate environment.

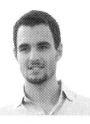

Short haircuts generally work for most men. However, extremely short hair is not a professional look. Certain short hairstyles such as the classic cut and casual texture work very well, as they require very little maintenance and still look good. Some styling gel may be required.

Medium length haircuts work very well in an office environment. Not only are such haircuts versatile, with the proper styling, you can pull off the "Corporate Elite" look. The most common medium hairstyles are the slick and formal looks. Simple styling

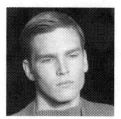

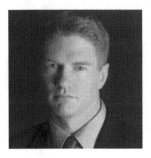

gel is used to define the look and in some cases, hairspray is used to lock in the look so that it does not fade.

Tips to healthy Hair

Have a blended juice consists of apple, banana and lemon daily.

Unceasing Impressions

The Importance

We have all heard the phrase "dress to impress" but most of us never heed the phrase in our work lives. In no way should office dressing ever be so simple nor should it be too complicated or provocative.

The clothes you wear reflect who you are as a person and your level of professionalism. Most business executives do not realize that professional attire commands respect, power and control. The most important rule is to respect the varying corporate cultures and occasions in your company. You are a "walking ambassador" and the message you carry can adversely affect your corporate brand.

Corporate Cultures and Occasions

Corporate Cultures

Every company requires a basic workplace dress code to typify the nature of its corporate culture. Astoundingly, these requirements are not reinforced down the line. Dress codes such as Corporate, Business Casual, Smart Casual, Casual Friday are unclear. The general narratives often recited by the Human Resource executives are appropriate, conservative, traditional, decent, presentable and comfortable. Service sectors are given uniforms to create unity and harmony and avoid individual perceptive mystification.

Corporate Occasions

The rapid pace of business today has led to a shift to combine business and social. People are more casual in meetings than previously. Occasions such as ceremonies, anniversaries, and annual parties are notable moments to celebrate. Dress for the occasion and raise your bar when you know what to wear and look discerning without being too sluggish. Classy, chic, refined and attractive professionals are ones who care for details such as fabric, right cuts, fit, well-pressed shirt and trousers, buffed shoes and accessories.

Male Business Attire

This section is primarily aimed at helping men attain a stylish, elegant and distinctive look.

Shirt

The first piece of your attire that is noticed is always your shirt. Wearing a well-fitting quality shirt can enhance the look. A tailored shirt conveys the attention-to-detail you, and every amount spent is a worthwhile investment. There are a variety of shirts that can be worn but they are usually classified into three categories.

1. **Plain**—These shirts are the most common shirts available and usually work with almost anything. An Oxford Shirt is formal. A dress shirt with French cuffs is smart, elegant and stylish. It is suitable to wear for formal events and even daily work wear.

2. **Stripes**—Vertical and pinstriped shirts have been a popular choice for many generations. Pinstripes provide an elongated look to the wearer, making them appear taller than they actually are. Pinstriped shirts are perceived as casual, as compared with the single-tone shirts.

3. **Checked**—Checked shirts are becoming increasingly popular due to their dual nature. A checked shirt actually looks professional and casual at the same time, which is the reason many people are starting to wear them.

Pants

The business pants colours are deep charcoal grey, navy blue and black. Black works well with almost every colour and the plain design of dress pants makes them suitable for any and all shirt types.

Professional Suit

Men's suits that are customized based on the body's measurements and proportions are costly but this investment makes an impeccable, polished and quality impression. When choosing a suit off-the-rack, a two-button suit is versatile. Ensure that the fine details are of a high quality. Such fine details include hand sewn seams and buttons, a symbol of good and fine finish.

Suits for Different Body Type

A single suit does not work on every body type. There are usually four different body types and hence four varieties of suits. These include:

- Petite Men (Below 168cm)—Single button jackets with a deep V will lengthen your torso

- Delicate Men—Double breasted jackets add a layer effect that makes the body appear fuller

- Heavy Men—Single or two-button European-cut suits will shape the torso, making it appear thinner. Deep V lapels also help to improve the effect

- Tall-Medium Men (180-188cm)—Three-button suits with a narrow V lapel work very well

Three Essentials Suit Colours

Navy blue is a great colour to choose for business suits. In many cases, navy blue suits work better than black suits. Deep grey suits are classier than black suits. However, it is not smarter to wear a tuxedo in shades other than white and black.

Accessories

The final options that have to be made are all the little accessories. These few accessories are usually combined with a suit to enhance the look it exudes. These accessories include:

- **Ties**—A silk tie is a formal accessory and is usually worn with a suit or shirt

- **Shoes**—Oxford lace-up shoes are more formal than loafers and are usually the ideal choice for most suits

- **Socks**—Dark coloured wool fabrics are durable for daily business wear. Keep your socks at above the calf length to avoid the faux pas of exposing hairy legs. Silk socks are made with fine fabrics and are suitable for very formal occasions

- **A Quality Pen**—Always have a high quality pen with you at all times, in your jacket pocket. A quality pen is a mark of respect, social status and success

- **Ring**—A ring is worn by many men, either when they are married or as a small extra. However, more than one ring may look awkward

- **Watch**—A quality Swiss watch personifies your style. Go with a genuine leather band for a formal, sleek finish. A silver band is functional and casual

- **Wallet**—Invest in a genuine leather wallet with two-fold flap. Only important cards, identity card, driver's license and cash go into the wallet. Do clear your receipts and avoid over-bulging, scrunched corners on the wallet

Female Business Attire

Female attire has become an area of concern in recent years due to the changes in female mentality and the perception of style.

In the baby-boomer age, the attire of most women was simple. The generation after them changed that look slightly to include an increased level of sophistication and professionalism.

The current generation has completely changed that look. According to the current generation, their look needs to be relaxed and trendy while maintaining a high level of refinement.

The first and foremost rule of female business attire is to never wear inappropriate clothes. Any attire deemed as inappropriate is usually revealing or tight-fitting in nature. They induce wandering eyes and are usually grounds for being viewed contemptuously.

Shirts should significantly conceal the bust and skirts, in case they are worn, should reach two fingers below or just above the knees.

The second rule is to never wear anything too casual. Women have a bigger choice in their attire as compared to men, as they have a number of accessories they can match with a large variety of clothes. These accessories include:

- **Heels**—Heels can be worn but should have a maximum height of 2.5 inches

- **Shoes**—Open toes shoes are casual and closed, pointed toes are formal

- **Hosiery**—Many women who wear skirts that reach above the knees usually wear hosiery with them. This creates a more sophisticated look

- **Skirts**—Pencil skirt suits are typically formal. Pant suits, however, are deemed casual on women

- **Dress**—A little black dress (LBD) works well in cocktail parties. The same dress with a blazer works best for office situations

- **Silk and Satin**—Choose fashionable fabrics like silk and satin of high quality.

Just like male attire, female attire should be kept professional and attract the least amount of unwanted attention. Always mix and match accessories and create a fab (not fashion), chic and in-control look.

Always ensure that you are well groomed, dressed and kempt. Never show a lazy and unprofessional attitude that could hinder your personal performance or inter-office relations.

The Power of Colors

Color Analysis is a set of color theory to define your dominant color in your skin—cool for blue undertone or warm for golden undertone. Once you know your skin undertone, you can determine your seasonal color.

How does colors affect your appearance?

What can you achieve through this theory? By determine your seasonal color, you can:

- Use your best complimentary colors for wardrobes that flatter you

- Time and money-saving proof for your shopping

- Apply mistake-proof makeup color palettes

- Use the color guidelines to mix and match the right accessories

- Discover complementing hues to your natural skin color for healthier and radiance.

- Invite positive aura energy and know your inner personality

- Create the extra glow in your eyes, face and hair

- Reduce imperfections such as eye circles, yellowish teeth, pigmentation, blemishes and uneven skin tone

How it all began

It went back to 1900s, Johannes Itten, born in Switzerland; a school art teacher developed his interest in geometric elements of the color wheel. With a few avant-garde artists in Weimar, Germany, he created the basic color theory. Under the influence and exposures from various artists such as Eugene Gillard, a Swiss painter, architect Henry van de Velde, Kandinsky and his halcyon days of art in Germany, Itten expanded upon the color wheel and invented a color circle with seven contrasting colors. He looked at every angle with creative elements of the psychological, psyche, physical, intensity and philosophic hues. Fast forward 50 years later, in 1950s Suzanne Caygill first practiced color analysis on women. This approach soon was innovated and promoted by image and color consultants worldwide.

Color analysis is a dollar-saving gift you can treat yourself to. Instead of wasting the amount of energy and time wandering around selecting the right colors, you knock it down with the power of confidence at the back of your mind. Shopping becomes a joy as you can better acquaint yourself into an array of your complimenting elements (accessories, clothes, makeup palettes, hair coloring, etc.).

"It is my fervent hope that we will all approach this new profession as a Behavioral Science. We must recognize that color does affect people's behavior through a deep sensibility to the psyche and its need"—Suzanne Caygill

The Suzanne Caygill Method

Suzanne Caygill is an analyst emphasize the importance of color, light, texture, pattern found in the face, hair and eyes. The basic seasonal group is Spring, Summer, Autumn and Winter.

The following chart is created for Asian Skin:

	SPRING	SUMMER	AUTUMN	WINTER
Color Ideology	Bright, Lively	Soft, Delicate	Rich, Warm	Strong, Dramatic
Skin	Warm with ivory, peach, golden undertone	Cool with rosy, pink, pale beige undertone	Warm with golden beige, golden brown, dark tan undertone	Cool with rosy beige, brown black, white beige undertone
Complementing Hair Colors	Toffee, Caramel, Dark Brown, Auburn, Copper, Light Chestnut, Strawberry Blonde, Golden Blonde	Toffee, Ash Blonde Copper, Cool brown, Platinum blonde, Soft gray	Red, Auburn, Golden Brown, Strawberry Blonde, Golden Brown, Chestnut Brown, Golden gray	Copper Red, Gray Blue, Fiery Red, Cherry Red, Aubergine, Dark Mahagony, Medium Chestnut
Metal	Yellow Gold	Pewter, Silver	Gold, Brass	Bright Silver, Chrome
Plastic	Tortoise Shell, camel, peach, soft bronze, pale turquoise, dark brown	Taupe, rose, blue-gray, clear	Tortoise Shell, Warm Dark Brown	Gray, Black, Dark Brown

Best Colors	Milk White, Chocolate Brown, Jade Green, Warm Pink, Camel, Tulip Red, Corals, Peach, Turquoise	Ivory, Soft white, Navy, Greyish blue, Rose Beige, Rashberry, Ocean Blue, Watermelon Red	Golden Brown, Moss Green, Mustard, Evergreen, Deep Charcoal, Teal Blue	True Blue, Black, Pure White, Fuschia, Ice Blue, Plum, True Red, Magenta, Chinese Blue
Personality Traits	Curious, Friendly, Witty, Optimistic, Energetic, Ageless, Hardworking and Independent	Gracious, Diplomatic, Gentle, Skilful, Practical, Efficient, Understanding, Organized	Decisive, Forthright, Loyal, Disciplined, Dependable, Earthy, Lovable, Individual	Poised, Elegant, Truthful, Sensitive, Creative, Ambitious, Self-efficacy, hardworking
Famous People	Kate Hudson, Jessica Simpson, Janet Jackson, Jackie Chan, Oprah Winfrey, Brad Pitt	Kevin Costner, Gwyneth Paltrow, Grace Kelly, Michelle Pfeiffer, Naomi Watts, Hugh Grant	Barrack Obama, Beyonce, Drew Barrymore, Jessica Alba, Kristin Kreuk, Kate Beckinsale	Audrey Hepburn, Katherine Zeta Jones, Lucy Liu, Sean Connery, Pierce Brosnan, Angelina Hutson

Summary

Appearance is beyond putting the right clothes on your physique. We lead a busy life, and we do not need a six-pack abs, neither do we live in a scraggy (stick-like) body. It is underneath the clothes that matter. You need to stay healthy and look after your skin and body. It is much easier for clothes to look good on someone who is in shape. Stay physically fit to keep your energy at the optimal level. This invisible aura can only be nurtured.

When you prioritize a healthy mind, you will constantly explore what is good for you. Eat at the right time and be conscious of what put into your mouth, how your body functions.

There is only one body, and you are living in it. You need to have a strong conviction on your intention that when you are well groomed, dressed and kempt, you are respecting the people and occasion. The Chinese proverb says, "there are no ugly persons but lazy people." The first impression is the last impression.

Chapter Two

Interview Etiquette & Dress Code

Interview Etiquette—Best Interview Practices

More often than not, you get the call for a job interview that's only a few days away and you start to panic. It is only natural to feel so, especially when jobs are so scarce. However, you do not need to fear, as the practices below will help you put your best foot forward.

Rule #1—Do not go unprepared

Make extra copies of your certificates, past compilations of work samples and prototypes. Arrange them in chronological order in a high quality black folder. Find good trusted references and alert them of your interview. Rehearse and practice your lines about your skills, experience and accomplishments to appear eloquent. The more credible you are, the more you win the smile from your interviewers.

Rule #2—Research

Find out more about the company's practices and the person who will be interviewing you. Take down his or her name and title accurately. It sounds familiar and warmth to hear his or her name used correctly.

Rule #3—Resume

Organize and print your resume on a high-quality, dense paper, also known as basic weight and grammage. Quality paper of 120 gsm signifies you value this job and demonstrates your personal worth. Have a twin-pocket portfolio folder in dark blue or black to take with you to the interview. The colour helps your resume stand out. Make extra copies of your resume with a cover letter. Sign your cover letter in blue ink, as it stands out from the sea of black printed words. Place it on the right and the resume on the left side of the opened folder. Prepare a letter of recommendation or reference and other additional documents underneath the resume in the order of precedence. Bring a small notebook and a decent pen with you to take important pointers. When you provide the documents in an organized manner, you impress the interviewer at first sight, stand out and are seen as a well-prepared candidate.

If you are uncertain of how to dress, visit your prospective company's website. There are bound to be pictures of current employees whom you can get an idea from.

Rule #4—Dress for your position

When it comes to dressing properly, most people spend hours trying to decide what to wear, what not to wear, what is appropriate, if you look too sophisticated or not professional enough, what tie you should match with the suit or even what heels to wear. These questions typically drive an interviewee insane. You will rarely see a CEO in casual attire, nor will you see a mailman wearing a top-notch business suit. It is important to know what position you are applying for and dress accordingly. If you are applying for a representative position, it is critical to look classy and refined.

However, there are a few short rules that you need to follow in order to alleviate your stress and ace the interview.

Business Formal vs. Business Casual

There are two types of business attire; business formal and business casual. Both are distinctive and both have an expert aura surrounding them. However, both do have certain differences. Below is a detailed look at what each of the two is and their differences.

What is Business Formal?

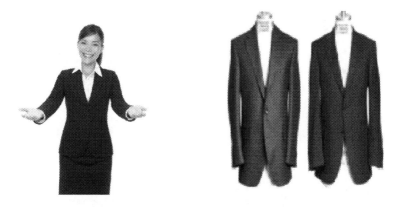

Business Formal is what you would normally wear to work. It is the attire of the corporate elites and is the clothes that really do make you look like a qualified specialist. Unlike business casual, your look should be sharp but not flashy. You should be able to radiate elegance without looking too formal. The whole idea is to display your specific persona rather than the clothes.

Formal business attire requires a suit, blouse, dress pant/skirt and shoes in a conservative and neutral colour like navy blue, charcoal grey, deep grey and black. For females, a skirt suit is recommended unless your research indicates that pant suits are acceptable in the company.

What is Business Casual?

Business casual is a more relaxed yet polished look. It balances the mild professional look and spices it up to create a look that is trendy yet sharp. There are a few guidelines to this look which you should adhere to so as to ensure that the overall look is business casual rather than casual.

These guidelines include:

- Wear dresses in ¾ sleeve or long sleeve and a pencil design bottom

- High-waisted blouse dresses in a single piece would prevent bunching at the waist and should therefore be preferred

- Well tailored conservative pencil skirts, pants, dresses and blazers are appropriate

- Urbanity and chic are encouraged but flashy patterns should be avoided. Small floral prints, high-cut splits, plunging necklines, short skirts, lacy & transparent blouses, clingy or revealing décolletages should be avoided

- Business casual does not mean you can wear whatever you want but rather stylizing formal wear to look sophisticated and smart.

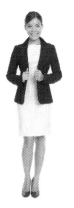

Style up your
Business Casual to
look sophisticated
and smart

Looking Your Best for Interview in Business Formal

The word "sharp" is best described on one that can pull out a **Business Formal suit**.

Guidelines on how to wear a Business Suit

Look out for shoulder seam that rested comfortably on the edge of your shoulder, arm holes that allow the range of motions. The shirt cuffs should display a half an inch access of your jacket. A narrowed waist-cut should make you slimmer and taller. The bottom of the jacket should not be too tight or flare out. The length of the jacket is measured where your finger knuckle is hanging down naturally. When you pair it with a pair of polished shoes and well-tailored trousers, you are aesthetically pleasing. Add your smile and a sleek hairstyle, your score is almost perfect!

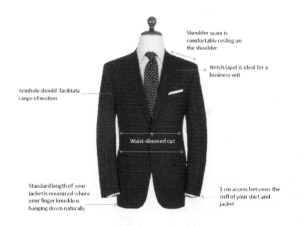

There are few tips that have been organized by category and relate to the upper and lower sections of the suit and also any accessories.

- Prioritize the navy blue suit, next a solid charcoal gray, followed by the subtle stripped or plaids versions of both colors. Black is your last choice (unless you are heading for a legal or hotel job).

- Although solid colors are terrific, stripes or light subtle plaids work just as well

Pants vs. Skirts

- A skirt suit is considered formal and should be worn most of the time

- Pant suits are appropriate for interviews with more relaxed organizations and generally for men.

- Skirts should reach the knee or just two fingers below it, as this will allow you to look fashionable without looking sleazy

- Pants should be tailored to fit without being extremely tight or loose and sloppy

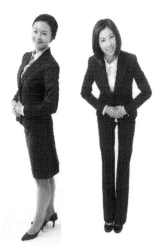

Skirt Suit is considered formal
versus the relaxed Pant Suit

Blouse and Dress Shirt

- Should be pressed, clean and well-tailored

- Solid white, ivory and soft blue are best

- Man's dress shirt to fit exquisitely for collar, arm holes and cuff length.

- Impeccable quality of fine cotton and crisp wrinkle-free

- Silk breathe better and are more comfortable in female blouse than other alternatives

- Camisoles can be worn under a jacket for ladies as long as they do not reveal any cleavage

- Avoid lacy, ruffled and glitter-like fabrics

Shoes and Heels

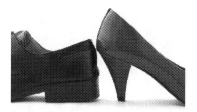

- Ladies—Conventional and moderate pumps

- Low heels are recommended (21/2" at most)

- Closed toe and flair or slim-flair heels work very well

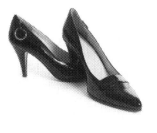

Closed and pointed toe with slim-flair 2.5 inches heels is highly recommended for business

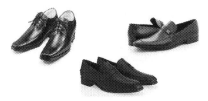

Choice of Men business shoes

- Men—Leather Oxford lace-up, Loafers and Monk strap are recommended

- Black and Charcoal Gray shoes work well with dark color suits

- Your shoes must harmonize with your suit's conservative tone

Undergarments

- A well-fitting bra should be worn at all times. Push-up or silicon adhesive bras should be avoided as they can add a slight provocative essence to your ensemble

- Use a natural skin-color bra rather than a black or luminous bra

- With a skirt, wearing pantyhose is suggested as long as they are skin-colored

- Shape-wear is an inner garment that conceals the love handles and supports your flabby butt. If you do not have confidence wearing a shift dress, the shape-wear can conceal your unwanted and protruding bumps

- For men who perspire profusely, go with a crew-neck undershirt in shades of light gray or white. They are meant to absorb the sweat and protect your shirts, a special name called "wifebeater"

Accessories

- Ladies—Jewellery should be minimal and delicate pearl collar necklace is understated, elegant and formal.

- A versatile laptop case

- A black folder and a quality pen

Looking Your Best for Interview in Business Casual

As with business formal, there are a few tips that will help blend casualness with formal wear to help you make your business casual look stylish and demure.

Pants/Skirts/Dresses

- Ladies—Conservative pants and dresses are acceptable

- A-line skirts, pencil skirts and shift dresses should be at knee length, though longer is acceptable

- Pants should be well tailored but not so exaggeratedly tight as to reveal the curves of the legs and hips

- Solid tones or subtle plaids are safer

- Avoid flashy, glittery, lacy and revealing fabrics

- Men—Pants' cuff should touch the sole. A single refined divot crease at the base when the pant collapses onto the shoes.

Shirts/Blouse/Blazers

- Ladies—Stay with long sleeves or 3/4 sleeves

- Men—Button down shirt, pinstripes, solid tones in shades of white and blue. A tie is compulsory and tuck in all your shirts. To stay creative and stylish, contrasting white collar and cuff adds taste to the conservative look. Short sleeve shirt has no place during interview

- Complement your collar with your face shape. Round face—pointed collar. Narrow face-spread collar

- Shirt and blouse fabrics should not cling the body

- Soft and neutral pastel colors are recommended. Subtle patterns can be included

- A dark color blazer is ideal for both genders

Shoes/Heels

- Very much similar to Business Formal for shoes/heels

- Closed toes and medium wedge heels can be worn. Peep toes heels can be worn for more relaxed business climate

- Avoid very high stilettos, scavengers, platform and groovy shoes

- Ladies—Match the style and color of your outfit with your bag

- Men—Match your belt color with your shoes.

Accessories

- Very much similar to Business Formal for accessories

- A leather dark file instead of a purse or colorful plastic folders

- Jewellery should be minimal and subtle

- A small diamond ear-stud can be worn. It should be in a simple design

- Clear-cut pendants, modest necklaces or other fine graceful chain necklaces can be worn

- Nude tone pantyhose are suggested for closed toes heels. Do not wear pantyhose with peep toe shoes.

Hair

- Should be neat, tidy and bun it. Do not draw any unwanted attention

- Hair styles with eye-skimming bangs reaching your eyelids should be avoided. Bangs should be at most just at the eyebrows.

- Avoid hair styles which excessively cover the face such as curly and funky layered hair

- Avoid spiked or bleached color hair

- Avoid tiny strands that stick out

Hand & Nails

- Wear only one simple colour or go without polish completely

- Always keep your hands moisturized as it is the first sign of aging

- Keep your finger nails short, clean and well-manicured

- A buffed shine is ideal. If you need to apply nail polish, go with pastel or transparent. Get a French manicure done. Avoid frosted, fanciful, dramatic nails and avoid nail art completely

Makeup and Perfume

- Be moderate with makeup and never over applied as you should exude a natural look

- Should not try any new foundation or two-way coverage powder to avoid any makeup disaster

- Choose a skin matching sheer foundation, blend well and complete with loose or pressed powder of the same shade

- Soft pink or peach blusher to compliment your skin undertone

- Neutral or creamy lipsticks should be the basis. Use lip balm rather than lip gloss

- Avoid clogging mascara or false eye lashes that make you look fake

- Consider avoiding strong perfume. To be on the safe side, avoid perfume and if needed, use deodorant.

Hide and Remove the Unwanted

* Hide tattoos and remove piercings from nose

It is better to be safe than sorry

In many cases, potential employees are still nervous and confused about what to wear, despite knowing the position they have applied for. Hence, it is better to dress formally rather than casually. It is almost impossible to dress just right, especially if you are nervous. Most people tend to under dress or overdress. Each look can work, and each can be salvaged in case the wrong choice was made.

When you are overdressed

Do not worry if you have overdressed, as this will convey a strong message about you and how serious you are about acquiring the position. If you are sincere, it will show and the interviewer will definitely see just how serious you are; this is called ambition. Most interviewers respect this fact and will admire you for it.

One necessary tip is to never remove your jacket and put it behind your chair as a lot of people tend to do. This action makes it look as if you assume the chair as a ready hanger and as if this is your office. It is a very rude action and should never be done. If you have overdressed, there is no need to correct yourself despite the onlookers. Maintain your poise, posture and confidence.

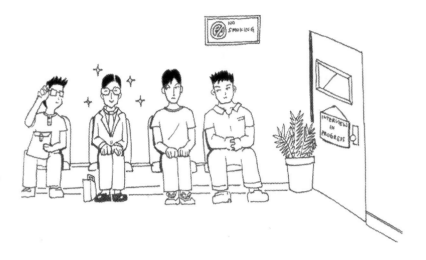

When you are Underdressed

If you underdressed, it is not the end of the world. Here are a few tips to make yourself seem professional despite the casual attire.

1. Maintain a professional demeanour to compensate for your informal attire

2. You may feel nervous but never let it show on your face or in your walk; walk and talk with professional grace while maintaining an erect posture

3. Speak formally and never colloquial your words

4. Button up your collar to be prim in a Polo-T shirt. Unfold your sleeves and button up the cuff. This will help to improve your professionalism and set the tone right

5. Always go with plain undertone long-sleeve shirt and dark colour pants. Do tuck in your shirt neatly

Anxious about your interview tomorrow?

The night before an important interview may affect your sleep. Have an early dinner. Make a green smoothie with carrots, celery stalks and romaine lettuce. These greens are high in calcium and contain calmative properties and tranquilizing effects to soothe the nerves. Practice deep breathing to ease away anxieties.

Interview Nuances™

You may now look the part but even your looks can only get you so far. Not only do you need to look like a proficient employee, you also need to act the part. There are three aspects of interview etiquette: body language, facial expressions and verbal conduct.

There are a few things that you need to remember:

- Always arrive at the office building thirty minutes prior to an interview. This gives you enough time to find decent parking, get directions to the office, fill in application forms and settle down.

- Arrive at the reception office at least fifteen minutes early.

- When offered a drink by the receptionist, turn it down unless you know you will be waiting for at least fifteen minutes.

- When the receptionist tells you to take a seat, given sufficient time; ask for the washroom if your appearance seems a tad off. Do not adjust any article of your attire at the reception.

- Always rearrange yourself in the washroom to check on your makeup and to just tidy yourself. The executive whom you are meeting should not let you wait for more than five minutes

- Always knock at the door moderately—two knocks with light pressure.

Body Language

Good body language is essential when you attend a job interview. The way you act and express yourself is as vital as what you say.

As the interviewee, you should sit on a chair which faces the door. This allows you to notice who enters the room, enabling you to immediately rise, greet the individual and introduce yourself. Make certain that you greet the interviewer with poise and introduce yourself the same way. Do not slouch or cross your legs.

Always place your briefcase on the right side of the chair (on the floor). Never place it on the desk or your lap. Your wrists or forearms, with the fingers loosely clasped, should be facing down on the table. Only your resume should ever be on the table.

The key to outstandingly refined body language is to glow with confidence. From the moment you walk into the room, it is crucial to convey self-assurance. Never underestimate yourself, as this feeling will echo through your body language. There are five key elements that must be committed to memory before your interview.

1. Give a firm handshake—A firm handshake will express how eager you are to acquire the job position. Never press too hard or too little.

2. Always maintain positive eye contact—The worst thing you could do is look elsewhere. The interviewer will immediately know that you are not focused and possibly not confident, you do not want to create the worst thought and cross an interviewer's mind. Do not let your eyes wander to the wrong place if your interviewer is a beautiful and a presentable lady. At an initial meeting, always keep your eyes towards her head. A great place to focus is at the forehead.

3. Keep your energy level up by sitting straight and remaining alert. Be optimistic, constructive and enthusiastic—tell-tale signs that you are pleasant and easy to work with.

4. Avoid being a chatterbox and keep the conversation flowing both ways. You should not come across as one-sided or dominating the communication.

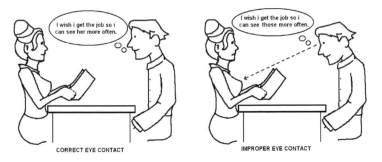

5. Never look at anything else, especially the wall behind her or at the rest of her body. Although this can happen, it should be watched out for and corrected quickly.

6. If you are being complimented, acknowledge it politely with a straight-forward "thank you". Never boast about your achievements, either.

7. Do not use a cute tone of voice or overly compliment the interviewer's looks, either. Flattery may impress her but will never be the reason you get the job. Play on your strengths and act as if she was just another male employer.

8. Remain enthusiastic and if you want the job, let it show through your words, your actions, your eye contact and even your smile.

9. At the end of the interview, rise up and push the chair back to the table gently. Take a few backward steps as you face the interviewer and bid farewell with a gentle bow. Face the door when you open and close it at all times. Small nuances do make the difference.

These facts are illustrated by the quote below:

If you have no confidence in self, you are twice defeated in the race of life. With confidence, you have won even before you have started.

—*Marcus Garvey*

Facial Expressions

Most potential employees realize how essential verbal control is but concentrating on verbal control alone is not enough. You will end up forgetting that actions speak louder than words. Your facial expressions speak more about you than anything you can ever say. You may say that you are confident in your abilities but if there is a nervous look on your face, your skills could be doubted.

There are two key facial actions that you need to control when in an interview. The first action relates to your smile. Turn the corner of your lips up while listening and mentally prepare for the correct answer. Avoid the "lizard-tongue" expression when you don't know the answer.

If you do not smile naturally, you may come off as a very insecure person. However, if you have an enthusiastic smile, your words and actions will have a greater impact. Always ensure that you nod your head to let the interviewer know that you are listening. Tilting your head slightly with the right ear towards the interviewer shows that you are an effective listener.

Those with nervous facial habits are prone to start frowning without even realizing it. If you have such a habit, make sure you keep it under control. Additionally, never scrunch your nose bridge or make funny facial expressions.

Verbal Conduct

Once you have learnt to control your facial expressions, you need to learn how to talk. The key element, as stated previously, is confidence. When you are confident, it is obvious from your words. The words coming out of your mouth will convey this fact.

For an interview to be successful, you need to prepare beforehand. Without the proper preparation, you will be mumbling and stuttering in the interview. Avoid having lots of Emm . . . Hmmm . . . Erh . . . and the like, as these word-gaps will communicate how unprepared you are.

To set yourself apart, always recite your lines at home in front of the mirror or in front of someone else. Script your lines and memorize some of the significant events and memories that shaped your profile, achievements and abilities.

This is your "selling" tool. Your words should flow fluidly, especially if you are nervous. Many interviewers utilize different interview techniques and tests, and never one standard test.

Some generic interview questions posted by the interviewers to test your capability, personality, experience, communication skills, business acumen, emotional quotient and salary:

Questions about Your Capability

- What are your strengths?

- What are your weaknesses?

- How do you handle stress and pressure?

- What are your qualifications, experience and how can you fit into this job?

- Tell us about your goals and whether you have achieved them or not?

- What do people often describe best about you?

Questions about Your Behaviour

In a behavioural Interviewing style, you will be probed and asked a few penetrating and sensitive questions. Here are some questions that your interviewer may ask:

- Give us an example of how you handle people who are resistant to change and how would you convince them that change is good.

- In your previous tenure, what were some of the initiatives, systems or changes you made and how did you go about executing those changes?

- Share with us some experience when you disagreed with a project and how you handled it.

Questions on how well you know about the Company

These are crucial questions to determine your desires and interest in the company. Find out more information about the people, products, achievements and cultures. Speak with conviction and admiration for the following reasons:

1) Your admiration of the Founder and recent news you have heard about his or her leadership.

2) How you are convinced by and trust in their products or services.

3) What are the impressive achievements the company has done?

4) You have heard of the corporate culture and habitat that you deem fit for your personality and work approach.

A stuttering, hesitant and mumbling interviewee will always be doubted. It is normal to feel nervous but it is unacceptable to show it in front of the interviewer. Always be prepared, despite the fact that you may or may not get the job.

Questions you should Avoid Asking or Discussing

1. During your first interview, avoid discussing and asking about your remuneration or pay package

2. Avoid discussing your domestic commitments. Never bring forward issues such as leaving early to pick up your children from school, why you cannot perform overtime, leaving work on specific days, any and all religious commitments, leaving work early on specific days to monitor your child's homework, going to extra-curricular activities, commuting issues; etc.

3. Avoid talking negatively about your current employer or complaining about the unhappiness of your past tenures. Furthermore, never speak negatively about your colleagues and any corporate policies. Do not grieve about your past employments. You may try to justify your frustration but may come across as unprofessional and negative. Worse, you may be regarded as xenophobic and lacking in physical and natural flair to handle challenges. Your business acumen is judged based on your positive rapport with your past colleagues and superiors.

4. Do not lie about your reasons for retrenchment or getting laid off. Be tactful and state the reason honestly for leaving your past tenure. Do not misguide your employer regarding your previous designation. This may work adversely for you when your potential employer conducts a reference check with your past employers.

5. Avoid talking about your health problems

- You cannot stand for too long due to a knee injury

- You cannot type for too long because of a carpal tunnel syndrome

- You cannot carry heavy loads due to a lower back injury

- You are allergic to some chemical

5 Intelligent Questions to ask

1. Ask about the job description and the specific skills required for it

2. Ask about the position and its associated career advancement opportunities

3. Ask about the expectations for the position, such as profit-sharing achievements, individual performance assessments, your reporting time and any subordinates

4. Ask about the management style and all immediate and future plans

5. After the interview, politely ask about the hiring process, the time span of your consideration and how you will be alerted to the final decision (and who makes it)

Agnes Koh

Summary

Below is a point-wise summary of this chapter. It includes some last-minute information that is vital to a successful interview. Also included are a few points that you should always remember.

ALWAYS:

- Dress in a simple and clean manner

- Wear appropriate under-garments and makeup that will not attract attention

- Wear plain shoes with closed heels

- Stay on the conservative formal side if you are uncertain of how to dress

- Be assertive

- Ensure you illustrate how unique you are and how indispensable you can become

- Always market yourself as well as possible

- Always talk in a friendly tone

NEVER:

- Wear anything sexy for an interview

- Wear any kind of knitted garment

- Dress in men's clothes (for women)

- Wear anything with a designer's name or logo visibly shown

- Wear a fake item or too trendy such as a "kawaii" look

- Wear anything too bold, bright or sharp in contrast

- Never talk about domestic issues

Last Minute Questions

- Did you prepare last night?

- Are your shoes clean and polished?

- Is your attire pressed?

- Is your hair well-groomed?

- Are you wearing any perfume? If you are, is it too strong?

- Are your fingernails trimmed?

- Are your jewellery and watch too flashy?

- Have you brushed your teeth?

- Is your breath fresh?

- Do you have an extra copy of your resume?

Chapter Three

Business Etiquette—Introductions, Manners and Office Decorum

Reception

The Receptionist

When you step into a large scale organization, the Receptionist's desk is the first place you visit. Many look past her roles and assume that she is a messenger who only needs to connect you to the person you will be seeing.

It is advisable to discern your initiative and, at the right time, politely engage in a short, friendly conversation with her. Keep the conversation short, so as not to occupy her time.

Regardless of your corporate rank, always take the time to greet the receptionist politely and ask how her day is. Although a small minute-long formality, it can make a huge difference to the receptionist's morale. As a receptionist, when someone approaches your desk, the following rules should be followed.

DO	DON'T
Greet in a friendly and polite tone	Be discourteous no matter how the dignitary treats you
Compliment their appearance	Neglect to pay a compliment
Courteously ask their name. Such an example would be "may I please know your name?"	Never ask "who are you?" or "what is your name"

| Look at their face (target the forehead) | Look at their body or what is in their hand |
| Ask them if they would like a drink, offer it to them and respectfully ask them to sit and wait | Tell them to get a glass of water or direct them to sit down and wait |

Importance of the Business Greeting

Some Quick Notes

You should always wait patiently for your dignitary to collect you. A rule of thumb for the dignitary is to not let your visitor wait more than 5 minutes. This is considered particularly impolite in Asian culture, especially aimed at people who are so busy that they keep their visitors waiting.

You need to respect your visitor's time especially if he has made time to travel to your office and meet you. Receive your visitor literally within minutes. Remember, lateness is putting yourself above of someone and disregard his time.

Receiving Decorum

When a visitor comes to your office, it is essential to greet him or her properly. Greeting plays a crucial role as it is the initial rapport building. It determines how approachable you are. It is, after all, the initial physical contact when both parties meet.

Ask them how their day has been and about any recent vacations, holidays or business trips they have been on. Additionally, you could ask them about their recent baby shower, family events, birthdays or the weekend with the family.

You may be surprised at what you may find out about the visitor. More importantly, you will find out how the visitor reacts and what "lingo" to use in your conversations with him/her.

When you are about to greet someone, you should follow the below protocol.

1. Stand one arm-length away from him/her

2. Square your shoulders

3. Maintain eye contact

4. Politely and naturally smile

5. Nimbly hand your business card to him/her

When you are a client and it is your first meeting, your business card is placed above the dignitary's card during the exchange. If you are a female of the same rank, you place your card above the gent.

In Asia, always hand the business card with both hands with a slight bow from the shoulder to pay differential treatment and respect to that person.

Giving a business card with one hand (American casual style) can be considered a serious offence and this will almost never impress anyone. Trust me, it is ill-mannered and will compromise your first impression.

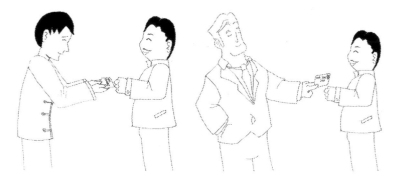

Always hand the business card with both hands with a slight bow from the shoulder.

Giving a business card with one hand is considered rude in Asia.

Greeting Protocol

The greeting protocol is comprised of four basic acts—the handshake, the ten-second line, small talk and the exit. Keep in mind that in Asian meet-and-greet culture, the handshake varies from internal, external, gender and rank of the audiences.

1. **The Handshake**—The handshake is the first step in the introduction protocol. Confidently extend your hand with a firm grip. Look towards the greeter and smile at them warmly while shaking the hand.

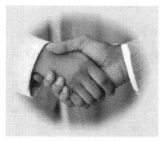

It is essential to keep your tone friendly and affirmative.

- If you are a guest greeting an office employee, regardless of hierarchy, always wait to be invited in and greeted

- Never shake hands with the colleagues that you see every day unless a special occasion arises

- In Muslim countries, most Muslim males add a slight bow and place their hands on their heart after the handshake. Avoid shaking hand with the Muslim female, unless she initiates.

- When two guests or new employees greet, the above rules do apply, with the exception of the religious rule

- A higher ranking employee should always be the first to acknowledge a simple nod, hello, eye contact with a lower ranking employee whenever possible

2. **The 10-second Line**—Create two sets of 10-second signature lines as a form of greeting. One set is for the initial meeting and the second set is how you greet those you are familiar with.

Many Asians tend to greet very abruptly or simply shy away with just their name. Greeting is a way of extending "Face Value" to the other party. Script and rehearse it until the 10-second line becomes second nature.

The 10-second-line is usually an exchange of names followed by "It's my pleasure to meet you". In case you are not new, always use a quick question such as "How are you doing?" or "How's your day?" This releases a caring aura around you and will necessitate a very short reply. This is an excellent start to small talk.

3. **Small Talk**—This usually continues from the ten-second line and does not last longer than 3 minutes. The small

talk notifies the other person that you acknowledge their presence and respect their existence.

Keep in mind that this is only an introduction and not a conversation. Networking professionals use small talk as an initial "appetizer" to establish a rapport. In Chinese, it is referred to as "Guanxi" (rapport and relationship building).

Prideful Chinese industrialists may feel totally offended if eye contact does not render down a minute "hello". Such Chinese industrialists will usually size you up and decide if you deserve any more of their time and effort and whether further investment into the business relationship is necessary or not.

4. **The Exit**—The exit has to be flawless and swift, otherwise the small talk stage will become a business conversation at work. Use an exit line such as "Allow me to excuse myself so I can . . . ." or "It's a pleasure meeting you. I enjoyed our conversation, have a pleasant day".

Introduction Protocol

There is usually going to be a need to introduce someone during your work life. It is imperative that you use the right address and introduce them properly. However, there are different ways to introduce different people.

Introducing an Employee to the Peers

When introducing an employee to another employee of the opposite sex, a smart move is to be honest. The aim is to give two people a chance to talk and establish a bridge between the two unknowns.

Introducing a Senior Employee to a Junior Employee

When introducing a junior employee to a senior employee, always address the senior first yourself. "Good morning/ afternoon/evening Mr. Smith, I would like you to meet our supervisor, Aaron Chan".

Turn to Aaron instantly and say "Aaron, please meet our President, Mr. Smith". This will demonstrate to the junior employee how to properly greet a senior employee. After the introduction, state the reason for the junior employee's visit.

Introducing Someone You are Familiar with First

When introducing a friend to someone you do not know, always state the person you are familiar with first and share brief information with the person you introduce to.

Introducing a Junior to a Senior

When introducing a younger employee to an older employee, state that he is younger but do not state the age. This will notify the younger employee to the fact that the person he/she is greeting is older than they are and needs to be shown respect.

When introducing an invited guest, always talk in a high, confident and powerful tone. If they have a designation (Dr, Ph.D.), state their name and surname first followed by the designation. If there is none, start with Mr., Mrs. or Ms. If you are unsure of a woman's marital status, use Ms. In Asian culture, the maiden name is used first. For example, Mrs. Susan-Lee Escrow as opposed to Mrs. Susan Escrow if she wishes to retain her own surname.

Office and Meeting Room Decorum

Just as you would properly act and behave at home or at a friend's home, the same needs to be observed in your office. Decorum is the correct word given to the behaviour and actions that need to be observed in the workplace.

Office Decorum

There are a few aspects of office decorum that are outlined to not only protect your personal and professional interests but also those of your colleagues. The aspects that comprise office decorum include:

- **Vocal volume**—When in the workplace, never draw unwanted attention to yourself. The biggest distraction is a noisy employee. You would find it very distracting if the colleague in your adjacent cubicle started making a lot of noise either by talking on the phone or with another colleague.

  You cannot expect others to not talk if you talk a lot. Only talk if you absolutely need to. If you do need to, talk in a slightly audible volume close to that of a whisper.

- **Always show reverence**—An age-old states, "Respect demands respect". Hence, it is quite clear how to gain and give respect in the workplace. If you want a colleague to have a high level of admiration for you, it goes without saying that you must be sensitive of how to treat them as well. This does not mean that you should expect to be given this appreciation first.

  In Asian culture, junior and young employees should show respect first. When being called by a superior, always knock on the door. Do not initiate any personal contact such as placing your arm over your superior's shoulders.

- **Be Modest**—It is crucial to maintain modesty in a work environment. The slightest immoral gesture could prove to be extremely problematic for all the parties involved. For example, neither men nor women should wear provocative clothing or wear clothes that outline the body and various features.

- **Keep Your Hands to Yourself**—Both sexes should rarely find the need to touch each other, especially in Muslim countries where contact between opposite sexes is looked down upon. The only case where it may even be needed is in the form of a handshake.

- **Keep Your Mobile Silent**—One of the most irritating things in any workplace is a ringing phone. It does not matter how important the call is, as long as you are on office hours, your full attention should be towards your work rather than your phone. That is, unless the nature of your work is highly reliant on mobility and emergency, such as fast turn-around services, sales professionals, call support staff, customer service, etc.

- **Refrain from Noise Pollution**—The open concept office has moved away from extinct cubicles to pre-assigned workstations. Keep your noise down when you are on the phone and lower the streaming music or wear a headset. Keep your phone ringtone just for your ear and assume that all business calls are important enough to pick each other's calls up and avoid letting the phone ring unattended. Avoid speaking in a belligerent manner to your colleagues when you need to discipline your subordinates. This will ease away any discomfort.

- **Avoid Making Personal Calls**—Your co-worker need not to know what time you will be picking up your kids at the nursery or what your husband dishes out for dinner.

- **Be Considerate**—Do not engage in a long discussion with your co-workers. Adjourn to a meeting room for groups of 3 co-workers, unless the meeting lasts for less than a few minutes.

- **Keep the Workstation Tidy**—How organized you are is reflected on your workstation. It reflects on your personal hygiene. Put away all documents when you are out for lunch or after work. Your table should look neat and clean without much decorative materials. If you must, display relevant materials of company events. Avoid too many personal artefacts, as you may not be taken seriously by others.

- **Keep to Yourself**—One of the fastest ways to get fired is to meddle in the affairs of a colleague. If a mobile or email is not yours, do not look through it. If it is not your computer screen, do not look at it. If you keep to yourself, there will never be any complaints.

- **Respect Company Property**—Never steal or borrow anything from the office, even if it is a small item. Ask first before you borrow even a simple pen from your colleague. Return after use to a central pool of stationeries. There are always cameras everywhere and you will get caught; it is not a matter of chance but time.

- **Lest I Wash your Mouth out with Soap**—Nobody likes an employee who uses foul language. Avoid using foul language at all times, even if you are angry. Even when in the company of very close friends, avoid using abusive words, as they can be heard by others.

Remember, you do not have to be famous for the wrong reason.

- **Office Romance**—Having an affair in the office is like setting a ticking bomb to your career in that company. This is excruciatingly serious if the other party is married.

Such relationships are never a sweet ride particularly if one party member is of a superior position. Jealousy, gossip, condescension and various complexities may cause prejudice against professional judgment.

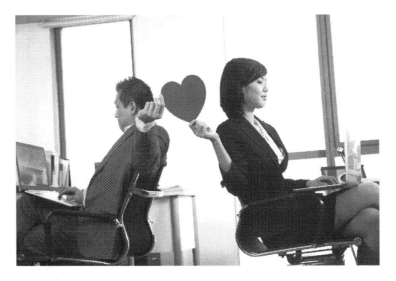

Office romance is excruciatingly serious if the other party is married

Meeting Room Etiquette

What you may not realize is that sitting in your cubicle is different from sitting in a meeting room. In a meeting room, for instance, you do not just sit anywhere you wish. There is a select pattern that must be followed. For example, only the CEO or the boss will sit at the "big chair". In an outward pattern, the normal office hierarchy is followed. The table below illustrates the fact; the numbers 1 to 8 illustrate how high they are on the office hierarchy where 1 is the highest.

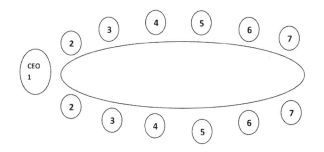

There are a few rules that must be adhered when in a meeting room, also. The foundations of meeting room etiquette start with the fact that you do not speak unless it is your turn.

Another crucial rule is that you never bring anything to eat or drink into a meeting room. If lunch is to be served in the meeting, you will be notified beforehand. If anything to drink or eat is offered within a meeting room, do not turn it down unless you are already full or have a good reason, as the gesture could be found displeasing, especially in various Asian cultures.

Always sit in a proper manner: straight, erect and feet flat on the floor. Never slouch, bend over, play with your chair or look around the room, as this is considered very ill-mannered.

Time management is also crucial. Attending a meeting late is considered very rude and dreadfully unprofessional. In your work-life, an unpunctual employee will always be unreliable and disorganized.

Technology Etiquette

Technology has changed rapidly over the years—more rapidly than we can keep up with. Technology has made its way into every aspect of life, even the office. With ever increasing means and platforms of communication, it is only natural that children and adults alike use them. However, when it comes to the workplace environment, there are a few rules that must be adhered to.

Social Network Etiquette

The social media era is being lived and it is not easy to turn away from the addiction that is Facebook, Twitter, LinkedIn and the like. When using these social networking sites, ensure that you do not use them during office hours, as they can become a huge distraction—particularly due to their addictive nature.

In addition, ensure that you do not mention office work, politics, religious discrimination, gossip or chat about private events on social networking sites, as you never really know who is connected to whom. It would be a shame to write bad things about your boss only to later find out he read it.

Facebook Etiquette

The number of Facebook users has risen to over 900 million worldwide at the time of writing, according to Facebook's report. People use Facebook to connect with their friends, keep up with news and events, upload unlimited pictures and chat with friends. Today, many users do not log out. With smart phones, they can update their status any time of the day. It has become a part of their way of life.

You can capitalize on social media tools to complement your professional network. A Facebook page is an excellent platform to promote your products and services. Think of how you want to present yourself and how your posts impact on the views of the readers, the frequency of your posts and how much time you spend to engage them.

For personal status feeds, do not over-post. You may end up being perceived as if you have no life other than virtual. Group your friend lists sensitively so you can select who can read your posts. Limit your vacation pictures to a maximum of 50 pictures. Honestly, your friends are too busy to sort through your 1000 pictures.

Your online existence calls forth vivid images within the mind of others. How you engage with others, and your "statuses" are reflections of how you would like to be perceived. Do separate your work and social groups. Assign your privacy level.

Good facebook etiquette is to watch over your response to "comments". When you wish to share a friend's posts, make sure you "LIKE" before you share. If you do not like to read something that your friend posted, simply ignore it. Avoid any foul comments. There are so many news feeds to entice you.

Twetiquette

When it comes to Twitter, these are the points to help you tweet more effectively.

No. 1—Know your lingo. The key terms and key words will help you optimize your usage.

No. 2—Know your hashtags. You don't want to use too little or overuse it. Two or three hashtags are appropriate numbers. Hashtags are great ways to signify key terms in your message.

No. 3—Engage your audience. You want to come across as a human and not automated. When people mention you or reply to you, they want to know if they can get a response back. Therefore, it is important to be prompt with your reply.

No. 4—Do not sell stuff on Twitter. You have 140 characters to add value to lives, link to cool stuff, give resources, make new friends and respond to people who follow you. Twitter is not a place to sell stuff immediately. Make them know you, trust you and love you. Then when you offer something, they will be more receptive.

No. 5—Don't retweet more than you tweet. Do not rely others to fill your twitter or be an echo chamber. Give credit where credit is due. Be sure to include the author or source of your tweet.

No. 6—Avoid obsessively promoting yourself for your business. People will quickly get tired of you if your tweets seem to be an advertisement of your business.

No. 7—Do not tweet unverified information. Rumors can spread like "viruses" on twitter.

No. 8—Do not tweet junk. Do you think your followers care when you check in at MacDonald's? It is a waste of bandwidth.

You will acquire a lot of followers when you add value and interesting tweets. You build relationships and you get a lot more from the twitter.

LinkedIn Etiquette

LinkedIn is used by people in occupation and companies, for job searching, hiring and by those who wish to build a professional network. It has to be authentic and upstanding. If you are in the industry of finance, recruiting, administration, you need a more professional-looking photo. If you are in an industry like art, advertising, creative or fashion, you can get away with a casual photo. Manage your profile like your resume. Keep your privacy setting so that your new connections do not get to see your past employment history. You would not like your other connections to know that you are job hunting.

Be professional in the virtual world. When your request for connection is accepted, it is polite to say Hello to the new connection as if you are meeting the person in business. Do not over-post on a professional networking site. It may appear that you are always out of your office and have nothing to do but empty entertainment.

Mobile Etiquette

During office hours, your full and undivided attention should be towards your work and not your phone. Silence your phone and avoid talking on it. One of the most irritating things is messaging within an office.

Many people seem to message their colleagues that are working only a few feet away. Although you are wasting your own time, the fact is that it is also distracting to them and due to their relation with you, they might not tell you.

Audio Etiquette

Office life may sometimes get boring and it's only natural that you look for other means of entertainment to help you relax or liven up. A good number of people listen to music during office hours to pass the time. The work of certain employees may rely on the use of audio files.

Regardless, if you need to listen to any audio in your office for whatever reason, ensure that only you listen to it. Do not increase the volume to a level where it is audible to others, as that is being inconsiderate.

Email Etiquette

A lot of communication in today's day and age is done via emails. An email is an electronic medium of mailing where the mail arrives almost instantly. When emailing friends, good grammar may not be a problem; however, when it comes to work-related emails, the proper use of grammar and the removal of slang, colloquialisms and general terms must be observed.

Never use any slang/colloquial words in an email, as it is deemed inappropriate. In addition, never use any emoticons, as it is not appropriate. You would never want your boss to send you an email stating "You are fired . . . LOL =P" as it is very unprofessional.

Social Etiquette

Special Words and Phrases

What most people do not realize is that the small things count a lot in the workplace. A simple "thank you" or compliment goes a long way. Not only does it help create a pleasurable atmosphere around the parties involved, it also helps to promote your image.

Below is a list of a few "magical" words, phrases and "icebreakers" that can help you be the most respected and liked colleague.

Words

- **Thank you**—More often than not, this simple phrase of gratitude is not given, especially among the current generation. It may not seem like much but a quick thank you acknowledges to the helper that you are grateful that they took the time out to help you. It may seem to be a formality to you but a simple thank you goes a long way.

- **Sorry**—They say that the bigger man is the one who apologizes and walks away. The age-old saying is true, except it can be applied to women, too. A simple "sorry" avoids any and all unnecessary arguments and saves a lot of time.

  In addition, in the eyes of the colleagues, the person apologizing, regardless of being wrong or not, will always be held in high esteem.

- **Please**—The age-old "say please" still holds high value in the millennium. A simple "please" before a question should always be used before or after a question/ request.

- **May I**—The word "may" goes hand in hand with the word "please". However, it is more commonly used when an action is needed. For example, "May I have this stapler?" or "May I sit here?" It is a sign of respect, as you requested permission before doing something.

Phrases

Certain phrases have different effects on different people and can be used practically anywhere. The phrases below however hold a high degree of significance in an office.

- **Would you mind?**—This phrase is often neglected by the current generation. Although most people will not say no to a question, it is a basic courtesy that you use this phrase before asking a question.

- **How are you?**—This simple question is a sign of adoration. It shows that you care for your colleague enough to use this phrase. This is a very common question that, although it's been replaced by more specific phrases, it is still commonly used

- **You're welcome**—This phrase is usually used as a reply to "thank you" It shows that you acknowledge your fellow colleague. This inviting phrase will also instil confidence within him/her and is especially beneficial for new employees

- **I am sorry to disturb you**—This phrase is used just before you need to interact with a fellow employee. It shows that the user acknowledges that you were busy and wanted to politely and respectfully draw your attention to them. In Asian culture specifically, this phrase is most commonly used when you interrupt an employee of a higher rank.

- **Excuse me**—When said politely, this phrase functions almost the same way that the above phrase does. However, this phrase is more casual than the previous phrase. In Asian culture, this phrase should never be used to interrupt higher ranked employees.

- **How are you feeling today?**—This specific question should be used when an employee was missing the day before or if you notice that the colleague is feeling unwell. It can also be used as an icebreaker when talking to a depressed colleague.

Compliments

A compliment is a global word/phrase used to acknowledge another individual's hard work or efforts. Many compliments that can be used outside the office can also be used inside the office, as long as they are appropriate. Below is a small list of common compliments that are used in the average office environment.

- You look charming today (specifically for women)

- You did a good job

- You look handsome today (specifically for men)

- That was so sweet of you

- That is a good [food item]

Icebreakers

Icebreakers are particularly important when it comes to new employees. The name comes from the tension seen in ice. The tension a new employee has on his first day of work is a prime example of where such phrases are needed. Most of these phrases should be used very carefully and at the right time, as you may end up looking like a fool if used incorrectly.

Many icebreakers can be used to initiate contact or small talk and bring the talking party out of an awkward silence period. These phrases are especially useful when time is not passing by during a break period, the most awkward silence period of all.

Below is a simple list of commonly used icebreakers along with explanations on when to use them.

- **Did you watch the charity show last night?**—This is usually used during the awkward silence period. It brings up a brand new topic without much effort. Automatically, one thing will lead to another.

- **What is working here like?**—This is a question that most employees ask current employees. Although they do not expect a bad response, it is a great technique to tackle a group of colleagues rather than an individual and blend in.

- **Complaining**—More often than not, many employees will complain about something that went wrong in their life. For new employees, try forming a statement into a question such as "Is the parking in this building really this bad?"

  This should, however, be used carefully if it is used in the form of a question. Only use it when you know a colleague or a group of colleagues are talking about the traffic or parking

- **Bold greeting**—However, the easiest and unfortunately the riskiest way to break the ice is to jump right in. Go up to a group of colleagues or an individual colleague and greet them with "Good morning/afternoon/evening, I am [name], nice to meet you." If executed correctly, it can prove to be more efficient than any other icebreaker.

Car Etiquette

Most countries follow the keep-right rule on the road and cars have their steering wheels on the left. Other countries like Japan, Australia, England, Singapore, Thailand, Indonesia, Malaysia and mostly Southeast Asia follow the keep-left rule. The steering wheel is on the right.

Car Seats' Precedence (Southeast Asia Context)

The driver's seat is situated on the right. The VIP is seated on the left curb side behind the passenger seat. Order of precedence is to allow the junior officers to enter the car, followed by the seniors. This would allow the senior to alight from the vehicle first, followed by the junior staff.

Entering the vehicle in order of gender

The female enters the vehicle first except:

a) When assistance is needed for handicap

b) In social and public areas

c) Rank takes precedence over gender

Social seating

a) Sit next to the driver if it is just you and the driver. You do not want to treat the driver as your chauffer.

b) The senior will sit next to the driver and the juniors are in the passenger seat.

c) It is polite for the man to open the door for the lady. Stretch your palm just above the lady's head to prevent an accidental knock on her head while entering the car.

d) Sit from your butt first and raise your legs together next while entering.

e) Always ensure that your shoes are clean. Right before you get in, sit from butt and brush by hitting your both feet to remove any dirt onto the ground.

f) If you commute regularly with someone who offers you a lift, it is a nice gesture to pay for the gas or top up the cash card. Do not take kindness for granted.

Train Etiquette

Public transport like mass rapid transit or metro in Asia is a daily clarion call for commuters. Dreadful and inconsiderate behaviors can make traveling experience uncomfortable. Some behaviors can be bad enough to make some civilized commuters act up immediately.

Do's and Don'ts when Riding a Train or Subway

Eating & Drinking

This is an understood social taboo that we don't even have to announce publicly. However, many commuters often discretely sip or reach out for small bites that cause a smell. To other passengers, it is frowned upon for not preserving and considering community courtesy as a whole.

Silent Your Phone and No Phone-Talk

A Japanese cute name called **"Manner Mode"** [マナーモード]". It means Silent Mode". Passengers are not to violate personal space in public. Keep the cell phone off when you are sitting within each other's proximity. Your fellow passengers will, at some degree, feel annoyed when you yak on the phone non-stop. Please be brief, lower your voice and end the call quickly.

Priority Seats

Giving up priority seat on trains is a social grace to the needy. In some countries, these seats are not occupied so they are available to passengers who are pregnant, parents with small children, elders and handicaps. Nowadays, there are so many thought-provoking voices on priority seats. Passengers who occupy these seats naturally "fall asleep" and often wake up by "self-entitled" priority passengers who feel they belong. It is saddened that this goodwill is taken for granted or disregarded. Everyone should naturally give up their seats as an act of kindness to the needy in the train; not just priority seats. It is important to thank the passengers who let you have the seat.

Queue, Wait & Alight

Wait with two separate lines for the train. Do not hog at the entrance door. Allow the departing passengers to get off the train first before you. Move quickly to the middle of the cabin and make room for others who are trying to get through the door during peak hours. Do not rest your back on the train holding bar.

Escalators

The unspoken rule on escalators is that you stand to the left while cruising. Anyone in a hurry could walk to the right. In some countries such as US & UK, the rule may reverse. Do not multi-task while you are cruising along these escalators. Reading and talking over the phone may slow down and inconvenient the public.

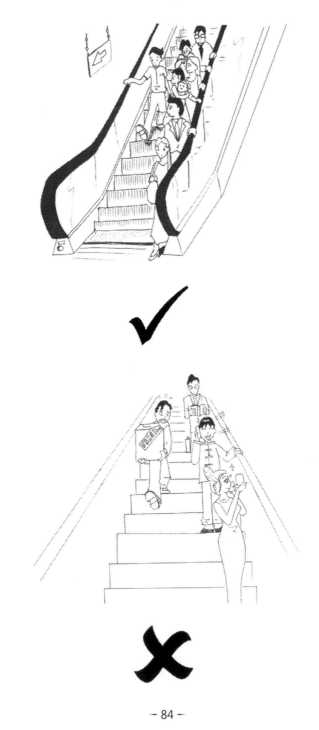

Receiving and Escorting the Dignitary

Chaperon, Escort or Military Assistant

The Chaperon, Escort or Military Assistant is a guide or companion whose role is to ensure propriety or restricted protocol in an important event.

a) At events such as inaugural ceremonies, occasions, exhibitions, site visits, balls, parades, swearing-in, luncheons, etc., where important guests are invited, the chaperons play these guided roles.

b) The chaperon/Escort/MA is detail-oriented. Every detail such as itinerary cannot be overlooked. It is a delicate role; the candidate has to be polished, presentable, intelligent-sounding, articulate, diplomatic and self-confident.

c) Addressing Protocol—Ensure that you remember the VIPs' titles, times of arrival, vehicle plate, purpose of the visit, and have the itinerary of the event at your fingertips.

d) Check if the main Host is present to welcome the VIP personally. You will need to lead the way.

e) Two groups of Chaperons—two in front and two at the back of the VIPs.

f) Arrival of the VIP—Open the door of the car, smile and greet the guest with a friendly smile and eye contact. If the Host is not present, you will assume the role of Host and extend the handshake.

g) Walk with the guest within 1 meter. Walk along the left of the guest. Always position a convenient walkway when it comes to an exhibition so the guest can browse through the show. Do not block the exhibitors or stand in the way.

Order of Precedence for Chaperon/Escort

Activity	Chaperon /Escort	VIP Gender	Protocol
Arrival of VIPs	2 Males	Male/Female	2 Chaperons Open both sides of the passenger doors for VIPs to alight. Or 1 Chaperon Open the left door and alight at the left curb side.
Departure of VIPs	2 Males	Male/Female	2 Chaperons Open both sides of the passenger doors for VIPs to enter the car. Or 1 Chaperon Open the left door and enter the car through the left curb side.

The Stairways

Activity	Chaperon /Escort	VIP Gender	Protocol
Walking Up the Stairs	Female	Male	Allow the VIP to walk up first
	Female	Female	Walk before the VIP and lead the way
	Male	Male	Allow the VIP to walk up first
	Male	Female	Walk before the VIP and lead the way
Walking Down the Stairs	Female	Male	Allow the VIP to walk down first
	Female	Female	Walk before the VIP and lead the way
	Male	Male	Allow the VIP to walk down first
	Male	Female	Walk before the VIP to lead the way

The Elevator

Activity	Chaperon /Escort	VIP Gender	Protocol
Enter The Elevator	Female	Male	Enter the elevator press the "Hold" button
	Female	Female	Hold the elevator door to let the VIP enter
	Male	Male	Hold the elevator door to let the VIP enter
	Male	Female	Hold the elevator door to let the VIP enter
Exit the Elevator	Female	Male	Exit first and press the "Hold" button
	Female	Female	Hold the elevator door to let the VIP exit
	Male	Male	Hold the elevator door to let the VIP exit
	Male	Female	Hold the elevator door to let the VIP exit

Gift Giving and Receiving

Gift giving and receiving is a fundamental part of business etiquette. During your work life, you will be required, at one time or another, to give or receive a gift.

When it comes to the corporate world, giving and receiving gifts is not easy, as there are many aspects that need to be examined and realized before any gift is made. Similarly, receiving a gift is not as easy as just a simple thank you. In addition, there are gifts that employees can give each other that a boss cannot give.

A corporate gift should be presented with no hidden agenda and is never personal. Giving a gift can help improve corporate relations and benefit both parties by enhancing their understanding of and confidence in each other.

Examples of where it is important to give a gift include baby showers, promotions, weddings, birthdays, funerals, farewells and holidays. The essential aspect of a gift is not the value it holds but the thought that was put into it and the fact that someone cared enough to give you a gift.

There are generally two categories of gifts that you can give: generic gifts and special gifts. Generic gifts include flowers, stationary, mugs, chocolates, cakes, cards and the like.

Special gifts are such that they portray a noble intention without being personal. Such gifts include magazines, spa vouchers, movie and event tickets, gift certificates, watches and pens.

However, these gifts and categories do not apply to everyone. Because of managerial politics, a superior cannot show favouritism and this is why most superiors give their juniors generic gifts. In addition, each gift has to be of equal or close value.

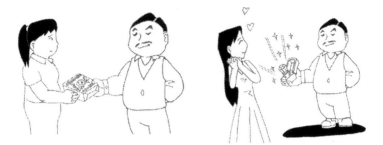

There are also differences when a male and female are given gifts. Cross-sex gifts can never show favouritism and can never entail a personal message. This proves to be very problematic. In the event of such a gift, politely turn it down by saying, "I think this is an inappropriate gift and hence cannot accept it."

Office Gifting

Office gift giving on social occasions is unavoidable. You will need to spend money on gifts. Gifts can be communal or individual. The rule is to never give a gift that you do not want to receive yourself. Do not give away something that you simply want to get rid of. You do not want to be perceived as insincere and thoughtless.

In a pool of many colleagues in your office, an acceptable budget should be $10-$20 for a casual colleague. You may wish to increase your budget to $50-$100 for close colleagues.

Generally, you can re-gift as long as the item is in mint condition and is not more than four months old. To avoid the same circle of friends knowing you are re-gifting, pass it on to someone outside the circle.

Spirit of Giving—Memento & Non-Generic

Special occasions call for a spirit of giving! A meaningful occasion is truly worthy of attention. Think about how you would delight the person receiving the gift. When you actually put some thought into the gifts, the feeling you receive when they open your gift will be of happiness. This is a memento. It is a sentiment and not unwanted clutter. Not everyone enjoys getting generic gifts such as chocolates, mugs, flowers, especially if it is anticipated and no longer a surprise.

You don't have to be the best gift giver, you can send a gift to patch a tension between you and your colleague. You can use this occasion to minimize personal differences and move on with a magnanimous heart.

Even communal gifts can be creative and personalized. Gifts such as home-made cookies, cupcakes, 3D cakes will be among your colleagues' favorites. Giving small token of appreciation to other colleagues not within your department is a good way to patch up animosity, misunderstandings, or grievances at work. You will not only salvage relationships but make your workplace harmonious. Please be discreet if you do not want to give a gift to a specific person.

If you are a manager or a boss, the best way to bond with your subordinates without showing favoritism is to treat them to a lunch talk. Often, I am invited as a speaker on Dining Etiquette at corporate luncheon or meaningful occasions. I must admit it is a delight to see their staff lightening up with fun. I can feel a special energy where they can learn and bond together in a social setting.

If you need to get generic gifts due to a large number of employees, always buy gifts of equivalent price tags:—movie tickets, meal and shopping vouchers, mugs, chocolates, cakes, cards and the like.

It is polite to ask if you may unwrap your gift. Never do so immediately, especially in Asia. Generally, if someone asks you to open your present in front of them and everyone, it shows that the giver has spent a lot of time, effort and money on it and hence is confident of seeing your joyous reaction. Opening the gift in front of a big group may embarrass and intimidate the givers who do not have deep pockets. Because of this, it is considered rude to do so in Asia.

Finally, if you want to buy a personal gift for your boss, try asking your colleagues if they would like to chip in and get a higher value group gift. If you must give a personal gift to your boss, give it privately without trying to impress. Make sure your gift does not constitute any obligation in return.

Gift-giving is an expression of love, respect and remembrance, try to be attentive, sincere and well-wishing in your gift ideas. Never give voucher redemptions that come with terms and conditions. Conditional gifts are inconsiderate. You would not want to buy something in order to get your gift. An authentic voucher is a cash voucher.

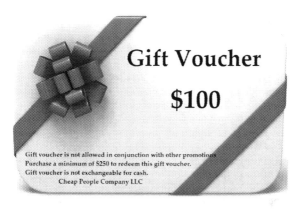

Gift voucher is not allowed in conjunction with other promotions
Purchase a minimum of $250 to redeem this gift voucher.
Gift voucher is not exchangeable for cash.
Cheap People Company LLC

Do not give voucher with terms and conditions

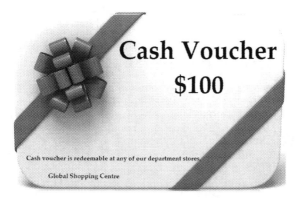

Cash voucher is redeemable at any of our department stores

Global Shopping Centre

Give genuine Cash Voucher

Chapter Four

Dining and Social Etiquette

Western Dining

Western dining and Eastern dining are two separate situations. The table arrangements, the meals and the style of eating are different. The most important aspect of either is to be a decent human being and observe proper etiquette.

The American dining style, in a nutshell, utilizes a *zigzag* style of utensil use. You use the knife, in your right hand, to cut the food while a fork is in your left hand. Once cut, the knife is placed down to the top rim of the plate and the fork is transferred to the right hand. Now you pick up the food with the fork, in your right hand, and take a bite. After the bite, the fork is transferred back to the left hand and the knife is picked up.

There are always many questions that seem to flood your mind during the dining experience. It is not the same for everyone, as there are usually different protocols for the guest, host and any VIPs.

You may have thought that you were going to have a good conversation and trade useful information for business purposes and ended up ruining it. Moreover, it does not matter whether you are a host or guest, Western dining etiquette must be observed at all costs; this is essential if you wish to climb up the corporate ladder.

Questions range from the mundane "what to order?" to the all important "which utensil do I use?" and each has a specific answer. Western dining etiquette is usually divided into categories that include, but are not limited to, table manners, ordering etiquette, guest and host etiquette and utensil etiquette.

- While waiting for the big group, look for your table name and place the napkin on your lap immediately when seated

- Never cut your bread roll but rather break it into bite-sized pieces. Spread the butter on one piece at a time and eat it individually.

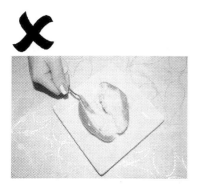 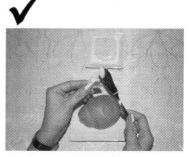

- Work the cutlery from outside in with each course. The "show-table cutleries" will be removed if you don't require them after the food is ordered

- Wait for the rest of the food to be served before eating. In a big group, the host would generally invite a small section of your group to start when the main courses have arrived. It is imperative that you pace yourself by eating slowly

- **Soup**—Scoop the soup away from you toward the north end of the plate and sip the soup from the side of the spoon. To prevent dripping, scrape the spoon at the rim of the bowl.

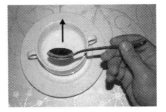

Continental Style—Use a fork with your left hand and a knife in your right hand. The fork is usually used to hold the food in place while the knife cuts all **poultry, fish or seafood**.

The fork is also used to pick up the food and transfer it into the mouth for Continental dining style.

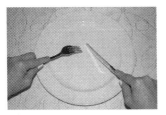
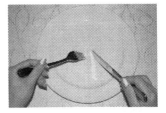

Hold your fork and knife in a sign of "7" position for meat dishes.

Hold your fork and knife like a "pen" when you have a Fish dish.

- **American Dining**—The food is usually cut into 2-3 small bite-sized pieces. The knife lays horizontally above the rim of the plate with the blade facing inwards. After cutting, transfer the fork to the right hand to pick up the food. Both dining styles are acceptable. It's better to use the style that your Host is using.

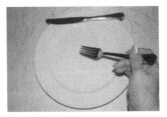

- *For **pasta and spaghetti,** use* a fork with your right hand and a spoon with your left. You can cut the long spaghetti; twirl a few strands with the help of the spoon.

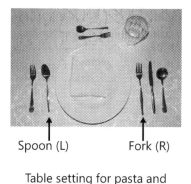

Spoon (L)   Fork (R)

Table setting for pasta and spaghetti

- While you are resting between courses, place your fork and knife at 5 & 7 o'clock positions with tines facing up. If you have finished and want to indicate so, place your fork and knife side by side at 6 & 12 o'clock positions.

- It is also acceptable to place them at an angle to the right (5 o'clock), as long as they are aligned together.

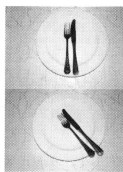

Meal Completion indication - 6 & 12 o'clock positions

Or at angle to the right at 5 o'clock and aligned together

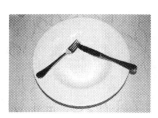

Resting between courses

Table Manners

Table manners are essential if you wish to remain at the table. Countless business deals may have gone wrong because proper table manners were not observed. Table manners are not hard to master and they are even easier to put into action.

Formal Western dining demands the table to be set in a precise manner. The pictures below illustrate how the table is set in a formal western setting.

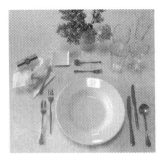

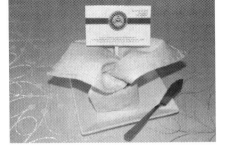

4-Course Setting   **Display of Guest Names**

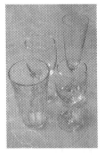

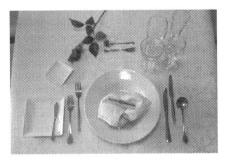

Display of drinking glasses   **Modern Setting**

The ordering etiquette in Western dining is different from that of Asian cultures. In Western dining, there are a few rules that need to be observed at the table. These rules are crucial for a successful dining experience.

- If you have been to a restaurant before, offer your suggestions.

- If your host makes a suggestion, never turn it down.

- If you want to turn it down, offer an alternative instead to be polite.

- Never order another dish until the other guests have done eating.

- In a business dinner, always let your superiors order first.

- If you have certain preferences, allergies or dislikes, let the host know beforehand rather than at the table.

- To remove any bones from your mouth, spit the item onto your fork and place it around the rim of the plate.

- Never pick up your piece in public as the gesture is very unsightly. If you need to do so, do it outside or away from prying eyes. Nowadays, the toothpicks' dispenser is available at the cashier and no longer display on the dining table.

- Hold a wine glass from the stem and never the top

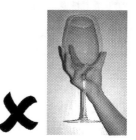 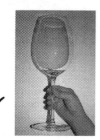

- Always use both hands to hold your napkin when dabbing the corner of your mouth. Never place the napkin back onto the table but rather in your lap

- Never use your mobile phone at the table. It does not matter how important the call is, you should never use it at the table, as this is considered awfully disrespectful. If you need to use your mobile phone, ask to be excused before receiving the call.

  Once a good distance away, answer your phone. However, in most situations, you will be surrounded by more people. Considering this fact, try to answer your phone outside the restaurant.

- Never talk with your mouth full, as this is one of the most grotesque things you can do and will surely leave an awful impression on the other guests.

- Never rest your cutlery with the food shoved in the tine. It shows you are greedy enough to worry someone might wipe up your food.

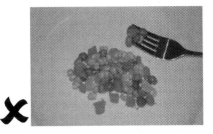

- Do not eat corn on the cob like a typewriter in a business dinner. Shred the kernels with your fork and knife. Add butter or pepper to the loose kernels.

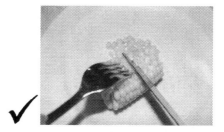

Another significant aspect you need to observe is seating arrangements. In different cultures, the seating arrangements usually depend on the event and the dining etiquette itself.

Guest vs. Host

When dining, there are subtle roles between a guest's and a host's dining etiquette. These small responsibilities may make all the difference between a successful dining experience and a complete failure. The table below compares the differences between a guest's and host's etiquette in a direct manner.

Host	Guest
Always reserve seats at a good quality restaurant you have previously been to	If you prefer a certain style or restaurant, make sure to let your host know
Makes a reservation in advance and always arrives 15 minutes before the guests do	Always arrives at least 10 minutes before the appointed time
Confirms the reservation a day before the meeting	RSVPs with the host beforehand and re-confirms their seat a day before the meeting
Finds out the preferences of the guest before the reservation is made and not at the table	Always notifies the host if he/ she has certain allergies or preferences
Allows the guest to order whatever they want	Orders a mid-range meal as courtesy

Make suggestions on what the guest should order based on your previous visits	If you prefer a different dish, politely use "I was thinking to order . . . instead"
Take your guest's order and convey it to the wait staff	Do not give your order directly unless you have been given permission to do so
Always ask the guests their order before the wait staff arrive and ensure that the chief guest is asked before the others	Always make up your mind on your order and let the host know what you will eat before the wait staff arrives

Southeast Asia Banquet Dining

Southeast Asia's banquet etiquette is built on tradition and not skillfulness. The Asians like to build on rapport, comfort and warmth hospitality. The traditions have not changed much. I would like to share my decades' experience in banquets, meetings, incentives, conventions and events in numerous deluxe hotels. I have put together these valuable insights.

Southeast Asia Banquet Seating Arrangement

Southeast Asia's banquet is arranged in a manner of superiority. Round table symbolizes unity. Long table represents ceremonial occasions. You can spot a VIP table by the red table cloth. In addition, if there are more than three tables in a Chinese Banquet, the order of precedence to differentiate the Host and VIP table are based on these three rules:

1) Right is the pride of place, as you enter through the door; the table on the right is the host table.

2) Furthermost from the door is a seat of superiority.

3) Facing the stage, the first table on the right is supreme where the VIPs are seated.

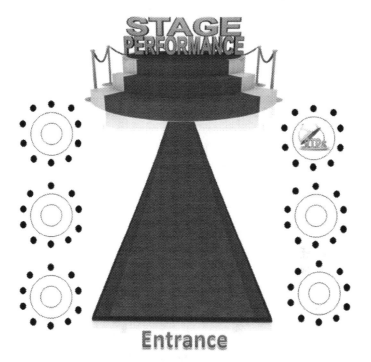

VIPs are allocated on the right furthermost from the door

Southeast Asia Banquet Seating Arrangement

There are visible differences between a round table setting and a long table setting. In a round table seating, the order of importance or rank of the VIP precedes. The Asian emphasizes "Face-Value" to acknowledge and respect a person's business and social position. Giving face is a way to distinguish the person superiority, seniority and partnership in a business banquet.

Seating the VIPs can be a challenge. You will need to know who's who besides the rank and title. Initial discussion with the liaising officer is crucial. Pride and honor are the key. At times, the liaising officer may be seated within the table. He/she may not hold a high rank but plays a significant role in the event.

Agnes Koh

Below are typical examples of round and long table seating arrangement for business setting.

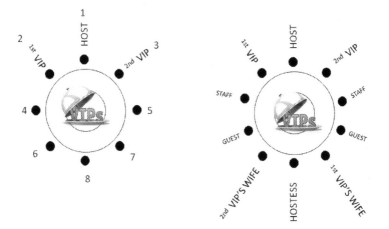

Southeast Asia Business & Social Banquet seating arrangement

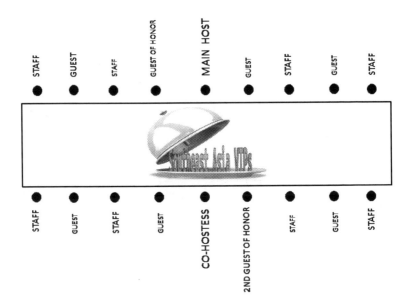

Hosting and Seating arrangement in Southeast Asia for VIP events

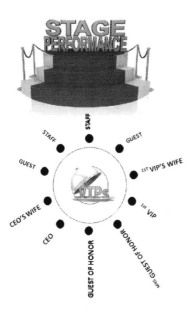

Seating arrangement for VIPs when there is a stage event

Arriving

Guest may arrive alone or with a companion. Always sit the ladies in order of precedence starting with senior in age for social function and senior in rank for a business event.

Women should thank the man and slowly sit with poise and grace. Remember to enter the seat from the left hand side of the chair rather than the right if it is a big banquet.

When you are arriving alone, always ensure that you talk to the usher rather than rush into the restaurant to greet other guests. Once you have been confirmed, follow the lead of the usher or waiter to your chair.

Leaving

When you plan to leave, try to ensure that you leave with all the other guests. If you are the host, ensure that you are the last to leave, either to pay the bill or out of general courtesy. Never rush to leave and never leave the table without excusing yourself first.

If you have to leave early, ensure that your host knows the reason. A host should never leave early unless there is a life-or-death emergency.

10 important Hosting & Entertaining Rules

There are a few important rules that must be observed when you are the host of a Chinese Banquet in a restaurant. These rules must be strictly observed, especially if your boss has asked you to host one, as he/she is testing your abilities and dining etiquette.

Rule #1—When guests arrive, ensure that you stand and greet them while they walk toward you. When a guest sits down, offer them a light drink or perhaps some Chinese tea.

Rule #2—Never snap your fingers or raise a finger in the air to get the attention of the staff. Wait to make eye contact with the service staff and request for assistance with a gentle wave.

Rule #3—Always use the wait staff's full name rather than "darling, honey, sweetie", etc.

Rule #4—Be polite to the wait staff and you will get an extra miles on food recommendation.

Rule #5—Dishes such as fish and crabs are charged by its weight. It is good to seek the assistance from the wait staff for adequate quantity, price and sufficiency.

Rule #6—When in doubt, go with the Chinese set menus. Most of the set menus are served in adequate portion from two persons to ten persons. You get to spend within your entertaining budget too.

Rule #7—If you are hosting, let your guest place the order first. The host will place the order last.

Rule #8—The dishes are communal. They are placed on a lazy susan in a round table setting. The guest of honour will be served first followed by the remaining guests, in order of gender. The Host is served last.

Rule #9—Never let your guests become bored. Always ensure that they are talking by asking questions, both personal (not too personal) and work-related.

Rule #10—Never pay the bill in front of the guests or let the guest pay for his or her meal, especially if the guest is an insistent payer. Excuse yourself and alert the cashier you are going to pay on your way out. Always pay the bill discreetly.

Being the Perfect Guest

Just as you would expect the host to follow certain rules and to behave in a certain manner, you should do the same. There are slight differences in being the host and being a guest. Below are a few points pertaining to dining etiquette that a guest should know.

- Where the host would normally arrive fifteen minutes early, the guests should arrive at least ten minutes early. This is to ensure that you never turn up before the host.

- When you are hosted by a female, treat her with the same respect you would give to a male host.

- Never leave the table without prior permission, as doing so is disrespectful. If you need to be excused, notify the host and wait for him/her to excuse you.

- If the host chooses to pay discreetly, do not wrangle over the bill. Do not commit a "diplomatic insult" to void the check so you could put the bill on your card. Be considerate to the restaurant's cashier and do not defy your Host's pride. Offer to pay the next round.

- It is cultural for guests to have several rounds of refusals before accepting the host's hospitality. It is acted out of modesty to maintain self-efficacy in Asia. If you are a foreigner, do not assume a candid "No," unless you want to lose your business.

- Do not refuse a drink. When you have to turn down an alcoholic drink, request for an alternative such as an orange juice or ice tea. It is a deviant act when you enter a restaurant without ordering anything.

- Sample each dish lightly so you are not filled up too soon. It is rude to stop eating in the midst of the feast. Your host will be offended and may feel unappreciated.

- Never start eating until the Host invites you to do so.

- If you have been to the restaurant before, make suggestions to the other guests but only if you know your suggestions will be preferred; otherwise remain polite and let the Host take precedence.

Chinese Table Manners

Resting your Chopsticks

Do not rest your chopsticks vertically in the rice as it is a symbol to pay respect to the decease. The two upright chopstick is reminiscent of the incense sticks and a sign of bad luck. Rest the chopsticks on the holder or horizontally across the bowl.

Do not turn over the fish

Fish is served as a whole in a Chinese restaurant. Remove the bones once you are done eating the tender top side. Fish is an auspicious dish in the Chinese tradition. It is a symbol of a boat load with fortune from the sea. You would not want the auspicious boat to capsize in business. In Cantonese, it means "turn over bones"—disloyal or traitorous.

Keep the tea refilled at all times

Traditionally, Chinese tea is free-flow and should not be allowed to run dry. The servers will always ensure that your cup is filled. You can tap the table next to your cup if you think you have enough to show thanks to the server and to cease pouring more.

Lazy Susan

Customary, the order of precedence in the Chinese tradition is to serve the best portion of fine delicacy to the senior members within the family or senior in rank (for business) followed by little children. This will help you turn the lazy Susan orderly. This respectful tradition has been observed for countless generations. It is polite to serve the person next to you, especially they are ladies. Do not turn the lazy Susan when another guest is not done picking up the dish.

Do not dig your "grave" and pick your "gold"

Do not drop the food back to the dish if you dislike it. It is unhygienic for salivated chopsticks to dig the dish and find the "gold." This is also known as 'digging gold' as a joke and 'digging grave' as an insult.

Red Packet

If you are invited to auspicious occasions such as wedding, baby shower, birthday of an elder; a red packet is mandatory. The amount ranges from a minimum of $100 to reciprocal value of your previous hosted occasions. The amount varies on how well you know the host.

Breakages

Asian avoids any breakages in an auspicious occasion. It bodes bad news and omen to the energy. Speak words of an auspicious proverb to void the bad omen immediately.

RSVP and do not be late!

It is generalized to speak of Asians rarely RSVP to invitation; neither do they show up to the banquet on time. Lateness is to put you above of others and do not respect the host. In a Chinese wedding banquet, many guests show up just minutes before the couple starts the march-in ceremony. The feasts are rushed through or a penalty charge for staff overtime wages to the host may occur. There are rooms to improve on this traditional faux pas. Cultivate good practice and arrive on time reflect well on you as a responsible guest.

Asian Superstitions

There are a few Asian traditions and customs that should be observed to avoid any offence to the rooted culture. A few superstitions are listed below.

- Giving a gift that represents fortune, luck, happiness, prosperity and wealth will bestow that blessing.

- Always offer condolences in the form of flowers and money and attend the funeral in person. Avoid wearing colourful clothes to the wake.

- To congratulate a colleague in the form of a gift, use red and colourful wrapping rather than dark colours or coarse bamboo paper (which looks like a joss paper).

- Never offer Chrysanthemums at auspicious occasions except as an expression of grief at a funeral. On the other hand, Chrysanthemums hold a place of honour in America.

- Never speak of bad luck or events that are related to misfortune.

- Give bracelets and anklets that make a clinging sound at baby showers, as this is a sign of prosperity, good fortune and happiness.

- Never give a clock as a gift, as it conveys to the receiver the message that their time is up. A homophone meaning applies to sending off the final journey in the funeral.

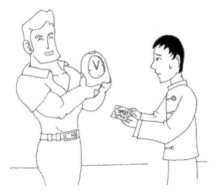

- Always remove your shoes when entering an Asian's home.

- Never go empty-handed when visiting someone's home; house gifts include food, fruits, pies or a gift focused towards a host's preference. If you are inviting a Chinese to your home, always offer a drink or refreshment as a welcome gesture.

- Never open a gift immediately, as it shows how "desperate", "hungry" and "uncultured" you are. When the giver requests for you to open the gift, do so graciously.

- Never overlook any auspicious occasions, particularly if the Host believes in "Feng Shui" and other aspects of wealth, luck and prosperity.

- Do not touch or allow your children to wander around any auspicious ornaments or move the office furniture. This may affect the wind of fortune entering the house/office.

Social Parties—How to Mix Business with Leisure and Mingle with Colleagues

Practically the hardest thing to do is successfully mix business with leisure. Consider the impact of your words and actions when you let your hair down too far. It may be a relaxed party, the Vice President and Senior Directors are observing. The conversations may perceived as casual, you are still in a business event. Never risk blending business with social. Do not talk and laugh harshly, dance like a bimbo or say frivolous things about someone; worst, flirting with your clients. Practice your best manners and exercise the power of "Mingling ACES" at every opportunity.

- **A—Amiable**—You need to mix into the environment as a warm, friendly and pleasant person

- **C—Cheerful**—You should treat the event like your own. Fill with good spirit to show that you are delighted to be part of it

- **E—Engaging**—Always be a great conversationalist who is always interesting to listen to

- **S—Smiles**—Never forget to smile, as a smile always radiates warmth and welcome.

In addition to the ACES, there are a few things you should also remember. If you do not know anyone, approach a large group of people that you may have seen at work. Politely introduce yourself and give a simple one line about yourself.

A great place to start mingling is the food and bar area. You can start talking to other guests while you get some refreshments.

Dos and Don'ts

There are certain aspects that should be observed while there are others that should be avoided. The table below summarizes the dos and don'ts of mingling. This table is the key to proper mingling. By following the table below, you can avoid embarrassment and enhance approachability, resulting in a successful mingling experience.

Dos	Don'ts
Always look your best	Attend the event in sloppy attire
Remain sober throughout the event	Never drink till you are drunk
Excuse yourself if you need to smoke	Never smoke in front of other people
Always arrive ahead of time by leaving early	Be late despite the traffic
Greet the host before anyone else	Waltz into the event without greeting the host
Gain permission from the host if you wish to bring a partner	Attend the event with a partner without asking for permission first
Tell your host you are attending the event at least a week in advance	Never RSVP at the last minute, as this is an awfully rude gesture
Plan the event well in advance and invite your guests two weeks in advance	Tell your guests a day before about an event. It is impolite and they may already have plans
Bring a gift for the host— Chocolates are ideal	Show up empty handed

Good Conversationalist vs. Bad Conversationalist

A good conversationalist has an innate ability to smooth out silent pauses and awkward situations. A bad conversationalist puts people off, contentious and condescending.

By reading the table below, you would want to put some thoughts about becoming a good conversationalist.

Good Conversationalist	Bad Conversationalist
Verbally generous with kind words, phrases and term of endearment	Miserly lip with few words such as "Yes," "No," "Think so," "Probably"
Sincere	Phony and conceal his or her real feeling
Honest and Conscious	Over indulgence of complimentary terms and effusive
Good Listener	Rambler who talk non-stop
Use words of Inclusiveness such as "Perhaps we can", "It may be of your best interest", "It could be a better suggestion"	All about "I", "Me" and "Myself"
Nothing to Prove. Secure and self-assured in what they have to say	One-Hand-Upper and want to prove his right of opinion.
No Hidden Agenda	Unsolicited advisor. They love to give their advices and aim to push a product to your nose.
Understanding and Compassionate	Chronic complainer, blant and insensitive
Bearer of Good news	Gossiper. Bearer of bad news and nose about others' privacy.

Final Thoughts

It is the final thought to reaffirm that business etiquette is the foundation on which your entire career is built on. Without good etiquette, you will never be able to advance up the corporate ladder. Do remember these final points.

- Always stay fit and healthy, as this will keep your body and mind active at work

- Always try to look your best without being casual

- Always keep your look professional and in line with your designation

- Always respect the boundaries of your colleagues, both in the office and outside of it

- "Work Hard, Play Hard". When you are working, stay focus and diligent. When you get a break, relax and enjoy as much as you want.

- Always carry yourself with pride, trust and credibility

- When in a party, do not get drunk

- Watch what you say and be a good conversationalist

And Finally . . .

It is my wish that you use this book in an advantageous way and learn something from it. I hope some of this advice proves to be an enhancement to your personal and professional life. One other thing is you may find some parts are common sense; ironically, many of you don't see these nuances coming through. It would be amazed at the number of CEOs who think the world is their oyster, but they hold the wrong fork, miss the "mark" and fumble at important occasions.

This book is named *Presence, Proficient, Professional* and the key to this is to practice till you make it. Keep shining with your grace and charm.

God bless you and wish you abundance of success in your undertakings.

About the Author

Drawing from her 25-year experience in the deluxe hotels and hospitality as well as her heavy involvement in Singapore's etiquette and wellness arena, Agnes Koh champions the importance of well-being in today's modern society. Her innate charm and soft skills are backed up admirably by an abundance of gumption.

Vastly qualified, Agnes graduated with a Bachelor of Arts (Hons) Business and Marketing at University of Portsmouth, UK. Her impressive credentials also include Certified Image Consultant and Certified Business Etiquette & Protocol Consultant from AICI CEU (Canada), Certified in Master Business Etiquette & Protocol from IBICA, Certified American Business Etiquette Trainer from ABETA, Certified Children Etiquette Trainer, at Florida, U.S., Certified Behavioural Consultant at IML, Inc. USA, and a Diploma in Holistic Wellness from C.H.Ed, UK.

Applying the knowledge and experience acquired through her academic and professional careers, Agnes injects her strong beliefs in honing etiquette, image and protocol skills into her work and designed programmes. To further advocate the social nuances, she founded Etiquette and Image International as an avenue to refine etiquette and image for school, work and life. She was resolved to promote a holistic wellness through specialized efforts in the various aspects of lifestyle.

On her first foray into the wellness consultation industry, Agnes followed an old truism: follow your passion in life. After all, it is this key ingredient that has led the highly sought-after etiquette and protocol coach to now preside over a team of associates and consultants to offer an expanded repertoire of services that marries her love for fashion and beauty with a unique combination of exercise, food science, nutrition and healthy living.

A recipient of the Promising SME 500 2014 Award by Small Medium Businesses Association (SMBA), Agnes is recognized across many industries to be a forefront leader on etiquette and protocol coaching. She raises a high cognition level in her consulting and is results-oriented when it comes to training.

Agnes believes an image is a psychological perception. Her testimonials have rooted her capacity to motivate her trainees with engaging and energetic teaching style. Throughout her career, she has also met eminent political figures such as the late President of Singapore, Minister Mentor, ministers and celebrities. She has also trained many MNCS and conglomerates and helped thousands of executives communicate their distinctive attributes through executive coaching and training programs, workshops and retreats.

For more than two decades, the company has established itself as the preferred choice of corporate clients to educate its staff on etiquette, protocol and decorum—its clients have recognized the value-added service and personal touch Agnes brings to the table.

Today, the brand is associated with the apex of holistic appeal: superior services, revolutionary concepts on social, mental, emotional, and physical wellness. Its mantra of "be the best that you can be " is also accompanied with a simple but sincere motto--"connect the world with etiquette." Agnes maintains the highest professionalism and adopts a conceptual approach when developing a slew of customized programmes. At the helm of the master trainer of the accredited Etiquette

Proficiency train-the-trainer certification program, Etiquette and Image International has seen great achievements.

As a strong believer of "the meaning of life is to give life a meaning," the wellness advocate is not one to rest on her laurels. She has published a children mannerism book to instill good manners and social courtesy in the younger generation. She is also a regular contributor to national print and social media. She has been featured, quoted, interviewed and shared her expertise on various aspects of etiquette, protocol and manners.

Far from merely running wellness, image and business etiquette consultancy, Agnes is also a passionate educator, cutting-edge entrepreneur, an exemplary businesswoman and a champion advocate of a holistic lifestyle. Selflessly promoting her noble cause, Agnes is a relentless one-woman crusader who will not stop until she is assured that every one has had a chance to pick up etiquette skills, starting from a tender age.

Acknowledgements

This book was written with a prayer manifested through our Lord Jesus Christ for His unmerited favors, supernatural blessings and unconditional love. One small favor is worth a thousand labors and thank you for living in me, for me and working through me. Amen!.

My thanks and dedication go to my hubby, Aaron Chan for his ardent support and tireless tender care. You always make sure I eat well. Thank you for embracing everything about me. Your affection and understanding are beyond words.

Special thanks to Stevenson Vdali Solkolov Tang, Shelly Edmunds and her production team for their efforts and contributions.

To you who have read the book, do acquire a mindset of a half-empty glass so you will have room to fill in more. Remember this quote: *"The World was my oyster but I used the wrong fork"* ~ Oscar Wide.

Lastly, Etiquette is more than understanding which fork to use. It is living with civility and treating people with dignity, respect and kindness regardless of hierarchy or beneficial importance.